NLN
PRESS

STATE-APPROVED SCHOOLS OF NURSING LPN/LVN 1998

Meeting Minimum Requirements Set by Law and Board Rules in the Various Jurisdictions

Fortieth Edition

JONES AND BARTLETT PUBLISHERS
Sudbury, Massachusetts
BOSTON   TORONTO   LONDON   SINGAPORE

World Headquarters

Jones and Bartlett Publishers
40 Tall Pine Drive
Sudbury, MA 01776
978-443-5000
800-832-0034
info@jbpub.com
www.jbpub.com

Jones and Bartlett Publishers International
Barb House, Barb Mews
London W6 7PA
UK

Jones and Bartlett Publishers Canada
P.O. Box 19020
Toronto, ON M5S 1X1
CANADA

[CIP data to come]

ISBN: 0-7637-0938-7

Printed in the United States of America
02 01 00 99 98   10 9 8 7 6 5 4 3 2 1

STATE-APPROVED
SCHOOLS OF NURSING
LPN/LVN 1998

Fortieth Edition

NLN RESEARCH UNIT

NLN Research Unit serves as a linking resource for nursing education and practice, research initiatives, community health care delivery, and information. For example, the Unit serves as a repository of nursing education statistics and maintains and expands NLN's national data bank, conducts research, and publishes results of surveys and studies.

Since 1953, NLN Research has been maintaining and updating a comprehensive data bank on all state-approved nursing education programs. NLN's Annual Survey is conducted using a sophisticated research design and rigorous data collection methodology. Every year, with the cooperation of each state board of nursing, NLN Research surveys the more than 3,000 nursing education programs in operation within the United States.

The NLN Research Unit is also exploring new opportunities to create a dialogue with members of the research community. To accomplish this, the Center has initiated the following programs:

Seminars—NLN has brought together intimate groups of major thinkers to discuss contemporary issues and set direction for policy, planning, and implementation. NLN's First Annual Research Institute held in August, 1995 focused on community-based nursing and public health. In 1996, NLN Research continued the series with the Second Annual Research Institute on the theme "Measuring, Monitoring, and Evaluating the Health of Our Diverse Populations."

Training—NLN welcomes pre- and post-doctoral students from the fields of nursing, sociology, psychology, and epidemiology. In addition, faculty visit on an ongoing basis from around the world. In 1995, NLN welcomed two faculty members from Thailand who received training in research methodology. In 1996, faculty from South Africa and England also visited.

Internships—NLN offers internships to provide meaningful research experiences that will foster the development of the next generation of health researchers. The interns have access to NLN Research's database, or they may use data which they have collected, to provide them with hands-on experience in statistical analysis.

In addition, the Unit has expanded into community-based research that is data driven and population-focused. Many of these special initiatives are collaborative, joining the Unit with partners from new arenas ranging from small communities to sister organizations across the globe.

For further information about other publications and activities available through the NLN Research Unit, call 800-669-1656, or use our internet address: nlninform@nln.org.

PREFACE

State-Approved Schools of Nursing—LPN/LVN 1998 presents the findings of NLN's Annual Survey of LPN/LVN Schools of Nursing, covering the period between August 1, 1996 and December 31, 1997. The publication provides a comprehensive directory of the over 1,000 licensed practical and vocational nursing programs in the U.S. (plus programs in the territories) with alphabetical state listings. A databank of information on schools of practical and vocational nursing in the U.S. is maintained by NLN and is updated each year by questionnaires sent to each state board of nursing. Each program is then sent a survey to collect the data reported in this directory. The directory lists all state-approved nursing programs preparing students for LPN/LVN licensure. For each school, the following information is included: address, telephone number, director, NLN accreditation status, state board approval, financial support, administrative control—as well as number of admissions, enrollments, and graduations. Unless otherwise indicated, all schools listed are state-approved. Newly opened programs and those that have recently closed are listed at the end of the directory.

Please note, footnotes are intended to help the reader understand some of the new options available to the contemporary nursing student as well as to clarify unusual features of some programs. A description of the footnotes appears on page x and it is suggested that you read it carefully.

A few schools have requested that the statistical information provided in the Annual Survey not be listed in the directory. This request has been honored in the school listings. The number of programs reported is based on information provided by the state boards of nursing.

A complete analysis of LPN/LVN data, including 10- to 20-year trends in nursing education statistics and data on men and minorities, appears in *Nursing DataSource*, Volume III, "Focus on Practical/Vocational Nursing," published annually. You might be interested in the other volumes in the *Nursing DataSource* series: Volume I, "Trends in Contemporary RN Nursing Education" and Volume II, "Leaders in the Making: Graduate Education in Nursing." In addition, the annual compendium, *Nursing Data Review*, includes findings from this and other NLN research projects including RN student and nursing faculty data.

Ruth D. Corcoran, Ed.D, RN
Chief Executive Officer
National League for Nursing

CONTENTS

JURISDICTIONS INCLUDED
IN THE GEOGRAPHIC REGIONS BY CODE NUMBERS

Region 1
North Atlantic

16 Connecticut
51 Delaware
59 District of Columbia
11 Maine
14 Massachusetts
12 New Hampshire
22 New Jersey
21 New York
23 Pennsylvania
15 Rhode Island
13 Vermont

Region 2
Midwest

33 Illinois
32 Indiana
42 Iowa
47 Kansas
34 Michigan
41 Minnesota
43 Missouri
46 Nebraska
44 North Dakota
31 Ohio
45 South Dakota
35 Wisconsin

Region 3
Southern

63 Alabama
73 Arkansas
04 Canal Zone
58 Florida
57 Georgia
61 Kentucky
71 Louisiana
52 Maryland
64 Mississippi
55 North Carolina
74 Oklahoma
05 Puerto Rico
56 South Carolina
62 Tennessee
72 Texas
98 Virgin Islands
53 Virginia
54 West Virginia

Region 4
Western

02 Alaska
94 American Samoa
85 Arizona
93 California
83 Colorado
89 Guam
01 Hawaii
88 Idaho
81 Montana
87 Nevada
84 New Mexico
92 Oregon
86 Utah
91 Washington
82 Wyoming

KEY TO ABBREVIATIONS AND SYMBOLS

Type of program (other than adult)
HS — High School
HSE — High school extended (includes high
school plus some additional preparation)

NLN accreditation as of January 31, 1998
A — Program accredited by the
National League for Nursing

Administrative control
SEC — Secondary school other than
trade or technical
TCH — Trade, technical or vocational
school or adult education center
COL — Senior college or university
CC — Junior or community college
HSP — Hospital
IND — Independent
GOV — Government agency other than hospital

Financial support (principal source)
PBL — Public
PVT — Private

Admission policies
Educational requirements for entering Adult program
10 — Tenth grade
11 — Eleventh grade
12 — Twelfth grade or GED

Other*
ADN — Associate Degree in Nursing
AVTI — Adult Vocational-Technical Institute
BOCES — Board of Cooperative Educational
Services
CETA — Comprehensive Employment and
Training Act
CLG — Closing
HOE — Health Occupation Education
HOP(C) — Health Occupation Program (Center)
HSC — Health Science Center
JTPA — Job Training and Placement Program
L.P.N. — Licensed Practical Nurse
L.V.N. — Licensed Vocational Nurse
MDT(A) — Manpower Development and Training
(Act)

Publication withheld—Permission to publish data withheld by school.

FOOTNOTES

NOTE: These footnotes are intended to clarify or explain some special features of some programs. They are not meant to be definite descriptions. Contact the school if you have additional questions.

ALL PROGRAMS HAVE FULL STATE BOARD APPROVAL UNLESS OTHERWISE INDICATED WITH FOOTNOTE.

1. Initial State Board approval.

2. Provisional State Board approval.

3. Experimental State Board approval.

5. For Army personnel only. As of this year, all Army programs throughout the nation will report under US Army Academy of Health Science, Ft. Houston, TX.

6. This program is currently inactive. Call school for more information.

7. This program is affiliated with an Associate Degree program. See State-Approved Schools of Nursing—RN.

SCHOOLS OFFERING PROGRAMS IN NURSING L.P.N./L.V.N. IN THE VARIOUS JURISDICTIONS

School Code	Name of School, Director of Program, and Phone Number	Street Address / City or Town and Zip Code		Footnotes	Type of Program	NLNAC Accreditation as of January 31, 1998	Administrative Control	Financial Support (principal source)	Number of Months in Program	Educational Requirements for Entering Adult Program	Enrollments as of October 15, 1997	Admissions Aug. 1, 1996 - July 31, 1997	Graduations Aug. 1, 1996 - July 31, 1997	Fall Admissions Aug. 1, 1997 - Dec. 31, 1997
	ALABAMA													
	23 Programs in 23 Schools													
023	AL Southern Comm College Mrs Margaret Denton, Chair *Chair's #: (334) 636-9642 Ext 658*	PO Box 489 Thomasville	36784				CC	PBL	12	12	86	126	62	43
026	Bessemer State Tech College Mrs Bobbie Daniel, Chair *Chair's #: (205) 428-6391 Ext 305*	PO Box 308 Bessemer	35020			A	TCH	PBL	15	10	156	177	68	42
025	Bevill State Comm College Mrs Alice Roberts, Asst Dean *Chair's #: (205) 648-3271 Ext 5430*	Drawer K PO Box 800 Sumiton	35148			A	CC	PBL			Publication withheld			
022	Bevill State Comm College Mrs Alice Roberts, Asst Dean *Chair's #: (205) 648-3271 Ext 5430*	Drawer 9 Highway 78 South Hamilton	35570			A	CC	PBL			Publication withheld			
007	Bishop State Comm College Mrs Deborah Connelly, Chair *Chair's #: (334) 405-4497*	1365 Dr Martin L King Ave Mobile	36603				CC	PBL			127	91	91	55
019	Central Al Comm Coll Dr Melenie Bolton, Dir *Chair's #: (205) 249-5716*	PO Box 389 Childersburg	35044				CC	PBL			Publication withheld			
037	Chattahoochee Valley St Comm College Mrs Dixie Peterson, Chair *Chair's #: (334) 291-4925*	2602 College Dr Phenix City	36867				CC	PBL	12	12	43	85	33	48
030	G C Wallace St Comm College Mrs Denise Elliott, Dir *Chair's #: (205) 352-8198*	PO Box 2000 Hanceville	35077				CC	PBL	12	12	72	70	40	72
018	G C Wallace St Comm College Dr Sheila Guidry, Dir *Chair's #: (334) 876-9338*	PO Drawer 1049 Selma	36701			A	CC	PBL	12	12	78	112	52	52
020	Gadsden State Comm College Ms Tarva N Vaughn, Coord *Chair's #: (205) 549-8683*	PO Box 227 Gadsden	35901				CC	PBL	15	12	84	96	71	57
006	Harry M Ayers State Tech College Mrs Linda Cater, Chair *Chair's #: (205) 835-5400 Ext 517*	PO Box 1647 1801 Coleman R Anniston	36201				TCH	PBL	15	12	127	91	91	55
015	J F Drake State Tech College Mrs Annice D Conaway, Dept Head *Chair's #: (205) 539-8161 Ext 129*	3421 Meridan St, N Huntsville	35811				TCH	PBL	12	12	77	102	69	70
008	John C Calhoun State Comm College Mrs Jane Floyd, Chair *Chair's #: (205) 306-2808 Ext 2808*	PO Box 2216 Decatur	35602		7		A	CC	PBL	12	12	72	96	52	46

School Code	Name of School, Director of Program, and Phone Number	Street Address / City or Town and Zip Code	Footnotes	Type of Program	NLNAC Accreditation as of January 31, 1998	Administrative Control	Financial Support (principal source)	Number of Months in Program	Educational Requirements for Entering Adult Program	Enrollments as of October 15, 1997	Admissions Aug. 1, 1996 - July 31, 1997	Graduations Aug. 1, 1996 - July 31, 1997	Fall Admissions Aug. 1, 1997 - Dec. 31, 1997
	ALABAMA												
	- Continued												
016	MacArthur State Tech College Mrs Sara M Goolsby, Chair Chair's #: (334) 493-3573 Ext 275	PO Box 910 1708 N Main Opp 36467				TCH	PBL	15	12	120	103	66	35
029	Northwest Shoal Comm Coll Mrs Suzie McCutcheon, Coord Chair's #: (205) 331-5200	PO Box 2545 Muscle Shoals 35660				TCH	PBL			Publication withheld			
024	Reid State Tech College Ms Patricia Gwin, Chair Chair's #: (334) 578-1313 Ext 124	PO Box 588 Evergreen 36401				TCH	PBL	15	12	142	164	87	57
009	Shelton State College Mrs Gladys David Hill, Dir Chair's #: (205) 391-2445 Ext 2265	202 Skyland Blvd Tuscaloosa 35405				CC	PBL	12	12	57	118	79	50
034	Southern Comm College Mrs Maggie K Antoine, Director Chair's #: (334) 727-3800	PO Box 668 Tuskegee 36083			A	TCH	PVT	12	12	46	41	20	23
011	Southern Union State Comm College Mrs Regina Beaird, Chair Chair's #: (334) 756-4151 Ext 5249	321 Fob James Drive Valley 36854				CC	PBL	12	12	53	71	63	22
027	Sparks State Tech College Mrs Sherry Barnes, Dir Chair's #: (334) 687-3543 Ext 273	PO Drawer 580 Eufaula 36072				TCH	PBL	12	12	50	44	28	43
028	Trenholm State Tech College PN Prog Mrs Annitta Love, Director Chair's #: (334) 240-9655 Ext 0655	1225 Air Base Blvd Montgomery 36108			A	TCH	PBL	15	12	138	273	74	120
005	Wallace College Dr Linda Parrish, Dir Chair's #: (334) 598-4598	512 Collinwood Dr Dothan 36303			A	CC	PBL	15	12	126	135	57	46
	ALASKA												
	1 Program in 1 School												
001	Univ of Alaska-Nursing Dept Dr Gerry Hansen, Director Chair's #: (801) 626-6833	510 Second Ave Fairbank 99701				CC	PVT	9		16	16	0	16
	AMERICAN SAMOA												
	1 Program in 1 School												
002	LBJ Tropical Med Center Mrs Toaga Seumalo, Dir Chair's #: (684) 633-1222 Ext 206	Pago Pago 96799				HSP	PVT			Publication withheld			

Explanation of footnotes on page x

School Code	Name of School, Director of Program, and Phone Number	Street Address, City or Town and Zip Code		Footnotes	Type of Program	NLNAC Accreditation as of January 31, 1998	Administrative Control	Financial Support (principal source)	Number of Months in Program	Educational Requirements for Entering Adult Program	Enrollments as of October 15, 1997	Admissions Aug. 1, 1996 - July 31, 1997	Graduations Aug. 1, 1996 - July 31, 1997	Fall Admissions Aug. 1, 1997 - Dec. 31, 1997
	ARIZONA													
	11 Programs in 12 Schools													
019	Arizona Western College Ms Judy Jondahl, Director *Chair's #: (520) 344-7798*	PO Box 929 Yuma	85364	7			CC	PBL	11	12	40	40	11	40
008	Central AZ College-Signal Peak Campus Dr Eleanor Strang, Director *Chair's #: (520) 426-4330 Ext 4331*	8470 N Overfield Rd Coolidge	85228	7			CC	PBL			Data reported w/AD prog			
005	Cochise College Mrs Susan Barnes, Coord *Chair's #: (520) 364-0216*	Douglas	85607	7			CC	PBL	0	10	50	60	0	60
011	Gateway Comm College (2 Branches) Mrs Frieda Muwakkil, Dir *Chair's #: (602) 392-5088*	PO Box 13349 Phoenix	85004				CC	PBL	8	12	105	109	77	59
018	Maricopa Skill Ctr Mrs Susanne Cook, Coord *Chair's #: (602) 238-4369*	1245 E Buckeye Rd Phoenix	85034				TCH	PBL			Publication withheld			
007	Mesa Comm College (2 Branches) Ms Claire Keyworth, Chair *Chair's #: (602) 461-7113*	1833 W Southern Ave Mesa	85202	7			CC	PBL			Data reported w/AD prog			
001	Metro Tech/Voc Inst of Phoenix Mrs Sharon A Pearce, Director *Chair's #: (602) 271-2650*	1900 W Thomas Rd Phoenix	85015		HS		SEC SEC	PBL PBL	9	12	0 34	0 40	0 23	0 40
009	Mohave Comm College Ms Lynn Young, Assoc Dean *Chair's #: (520) 757-0863*	1971 Jagerson Ave Kingman	86401	7			CC	PBL			Data reported w/AD prog			
016	Phoenix College Dr Daniel Tetting, Chair *Chair's #: (602) 285-7128*	1202 West Thomas Rd Phoenix	85013	7			CC	PBL			Data reported w/AD prog			
013	Pima Comm College Ms Vonnie Erickson, Dir *Chair's #: (520) 206-6661*	2202 W Anklam Rd Tucson	85709				CC	PBL	9	12	28	67	51	30
010	Pima Comm College Mrs Emelia Lewis, Coord *Chair's #: (520) 206-5140*	5901 So Calle Santa Cruz Tucson	85709				CC	PBL	12	12	63	62	45	27
015	Yavapai College Dr Lynn Nugent, Div Chair *Chair's #: (602) 445-7300*	1100 East Sheldon St Prescott	86301	7			CC	PBL			Data reported w/AD prog			

School Code	Name of School, Director of Program, and Phone Number	Street Address / City or Town and Zip Code		Footnotes	Type of Program	NLNAC Accreditation as of January 31, 1998	Administrative Control	Financial Support (principal source)	Number of Months in Program	Educational Requirements for Entering Adult Program	Enrollments as of October 15, 1997	Admissions Aug. 1, 1996 - July 31, 1997	Graduations Aug. 1, 1996 - July 31, 1997	Fall Admissions Aug. 1, 1997 - Dec. 31, 1997
	ARKANSAS													
	28 Programs in 28 Schools													
017	Arkansas Valley Tech Inst Ms Elizabeth Pruitt, Chair *Chair's #: (501) 667-2117*	PO Box 17000 Fort Smith	72917				TCH	PBL			Publication withheld			
052	ASU Mt Home Miss Victoria Oxner, Chair *Chair's #: (870) 425-3949 Ext 234*	213 E 6th St Mt Home	72653				CC	PBL			Publication withheld			
031	ASU-Beebe/Newport Mrs Paulette White, Chair *Chair's #: (501) 523-8966 Ext 0020*	PO Box 1120 Newport	72112				CC	PBL			Publication withheld			
002	Baptist Sch of PN Dr Shirlene Harris, Dir *Chair's #: (501) 202-7402 Ext 7433*	11900 Colonel Glenn Rd Little Rock	72210			A	HSP	PVT	12	12	63	89	59	0
030	Black River Tech Coll Ms Loretta Dismang, Chair *Chair's #: (870) 892-4565 Ext 256*	PO Box 468 Pocahontas	72455				CC	PBL	18	12	42	24	18	24
032	Cossatot Tech Coll Mrs Kay Lockard, Chair *Chair's #: (501) 584-4471 Ext 26*	PO Box 960 DeQueen	71832				TCH	PBL			Publication withheld			
029	Cotton Boll Tech Inst Mrs Nellie M Bowman, Chair *Chair's #: (870) 763-1486*	PO Box 36 Burdette	72321				TCH	PBL	11	12	44	44	31	45
014	Crowley's Ridge Tech Inst Mrs Gay Yarbro, Chair *Chair's #: (870) 391-3369 Ext 19*	PO Box 925 Forrest City	72335				TCH	PBL			Publication withheld			
004	Delta Tech Inst Mrs Kathleen Brewer, Chair *Chair's #: (870) 932-2176*	2916 Willow Rd Jonesboro	72401				TCH	PBL	11	12	42	49	48	22
022	Foothills Tech Inst Ms Gail Burton, Chair *Chair's #: (501) 268-6191 Ext 56*	1800 E Moore Ave Searcy	72143				TCH	PBL	11	12	22	23	22	23
041	Forest Echoes Tech Inst Ms Sheila Upshaw, Chair *Chair's #: (870) 364-6414*	1326 Highway 52 W Crossett	71635				TCH	PBL			6	12	6	7
011	Gateway Tech College Ms Geneva Taylor, Chair *Chair's #: (501) 793-7581 Ext 24*	PO Box 3350 Batesville	72501				TCH	PBL			Publication withheld			
035	Great Rivers Vo Tech School Ms D Boyter Evans, Chair *Chair's #: (870) 222-5360 Ext 222*	PO Box 747 McGehee	71654				TCH	PBL	12	12	29	25	21	30

Explanation of footnotes on page x

School Code	Name of School, Director of Program, and Phone Number	Street Address / City or Town and Zip Code		Footnotes	Type of Program	NLNAC Accreditation as of January 31, 1998	Administrative Control	Financial Support (principal source)	Number of Months in Program	Educational Requirements for Entering Adult Program	Enrollments as of October 15, 1997	Admissions Aug. 1, 1996 - July 31, 1997	Graduations Aug. 1, 1996 - July 31, 1997	Fall Admissions Aug. 1, 1997 - Dec. 31, 1997
	ARKANSAS													
	- Continued													
042	Mid-South Comm College Mrs Gale Allen, Chair *Chair's #: (501) 733-6773*	PO Box 2067 West Memphis	72301				CC	PBL			Publication withheld			
013	North Arkansas College Mrs Mary Wallace, Dir *Chair's #: (870) 391-3369*	Pioneer Ridge Harrison	72602			A	TCH	PBL	11	12	31	34	20	22
009	Northwest Tech Inst Mrs Ruth Jones, Chair *Chair's #: (501) 751-8824 Ext 112*	709 S Old Missouri Rd Springdale	72765				TCH	PBL			45	51	36	48
037	Ouachita Tech College Ms Lynette Smith, Chair *Chair's #: (501) 332-3658 Ext 52*	PO Box 816 Malvern	72104				TCH	PBL	12	12	20	30	24	20
028	Ozarka Tech College Ms Kitty Smith, Chair *Chair's #: (870) 368-7371 Ext 325*	PO Box 10 Melbourne	72556				TCH	PBL	15	12	32	18	19	15
016	Petit Jean Tech College Ms Carol Loyd, Chair *Chair's #: (501) 354-2465*	#1 Bruce Morrilton	72110				TCH	PBL			Publication withheld			
033	Phillips Comm Coll/U of ADEWH Mrs Cheryl L Hornbeck, Chair *Chair's #: (501) 946-3506 Ext 35*	PO Box 427 Dewitt	72042				CC	PBL			Publication withheld			
001	Pulaski Tech Coll Ms Sherry Bowman, Dir *Chair's #: (501) 771-1000 Ext 35*	3000 W Scenic Rd N Little Rock	72118				TCH	PBL			Publication withheld			
008	Quapaw Tech Inst Miss Betty Haygood, Chair *Chair's #: (501) 767-9314 Ext 352*	PO Box 3950 200 Mid America Hot Springs	71914				TCH	PBL			Publication withheld			
034	Rich Mountain Comm College PN Prog Mrs Charla Hollin, Dir *Chair's #: (501) 394-7622 Ext 1366*	1100 Bush St Mena	71953				CC	PBL	11	12	19	24	19	20
051	SAU Tech Mrs Mary Adams, Chair *Chair's #: (870) 574-4585*	100 Carr Rd E Camden	71701				CC	PBL	10		23	30	18	27
019	South Ark Comm College Miss Betty F Owen, Chair *Chair's #: (870) 864-7118 Ext 234*	PO Box 7010 El Dorado	71731				CC	PBL	11	12	53	54	51	27
006	Southeast AR Tech College Mrs Diann W Williams, Coord *Chair's #: (870) 543-5929*	1900 Hazel St Pine Bluff	71603				TCH	PBL	11	12	63	63	52	0

School Code	Name of School, Director of Program, and Phone Number	Street Address / City or Town and Zip Code	Footnotes	Type of Program	NLNAC Accreditation as of January 31, 1998	Administrative Control	Financial Support (principal source)	Number of Months in Program	Educational Requirements for Entering Adult Program	Enrollments as of October 15, 1997	Admissions Aug. 1, 1996 - July 31, 1997	Graduations Aug. 1, 1996 - July 31, 1997	Fall Admissions Aug. 1, 1997 - Dec. 31, 1997
	ARKANSAS **- Continued**												
020	Univ of AR Comm Coll Mrs Laura Massey, Chair *Chair's #: (870) 777-5722 Ext 278*	PO Box 140 Hwy 295 Hope 71801				CC	PBL	18	12	24	0	21	26
010	Westark Comm College PN Prog Ms Kathy J Redding, Dir *Chair's #: (501) 788-7376*	Box 3649 Fort Smith 72913				CC	PBL	12	12	20	44	15	22
	CALIFORNIA **86 Programs in 74 Schools**												
089	Allan Hancock College Ms Ellen White, Dir *Chair's #: (805) 922-6966 Ext 3383*	800 S College Dr Santa Maria 93454				CC	PBL			Publication withheld			
023	American Career College Mrs Diane Neville, Dir *Chair's #: (213) 668-7555 Ext 207*	4021 Rosewood Ave Los Angeles 90004				TCH	PVT			Publication withheld			
047	Antelope Valley College Dr Vivian Thornton, Dean *Chair's #: (805) 722-6402*	3041 W Avenue K Lancaster 93536	7			CC	PBL	0		15	15	12	0
004	Bakersfield College-Dept of Nsg, Ms Sheran DeLeon, Dir *Chair's #: (805) 395-4281*	1801 Panorama Dr Bakersfield 93305				CC	PBL	18	12	34	45	17	0
087	Butte Jr College Dist Ms Linda L Clark, Chair *Chair's #: (530) 895-2329*	3536 Butte Campus Dr Oroville 95965				CC	PBL	18	12	45	48	20	0
053	Cabrillo College-VN Dept Mrs Joan Frommhagern, Dir *Chair's #: (408) 479-6280*	6500 Soquel Dr Aptos 95003				CC	PBL			Publication withheld			
716	Casa Loma College (2 Campuses) Ms Maryann Frauenholz, Director *Chair's #: (213) 290-6440*	14445 Olive View Dr Sylmar 91342			A	TCH	PVT	12	12	133	179	167	39
733	Central County Occup Ctr Ms Meg Stanley, Director *Chair's #: (408) 723-6400 Ext 509*	760 Hillsdale Ave San Jose 95136				TCH	PBL			Publication withheld			
728	Cerro Coso Comm College Ms Mary T Kowalski, Dir *Chair's #: (760) 384-6333*	3000 College Heights Blvd Ridgecrest 93555				CC	PBL			Publication withheld			
024	Chaffey College Mrs S Gray-Dawson, Dir *Chair's #: (909) 941-2695*	5885 Haven Ave Rancho Cucamonga 91701				CC	PBL			Publication withheld			

Explanation of footnotes on page x

School Code	Name of School, Director of Program, and Phone Number	Street Address, City or Town and Zip Code	Footnotes	Type of Program	NLNAC Accreditation as of January 31, 1998	Administrative Control	Financial Support (principal source)	Number of Months in Program	Educational Requirements for Entering Adult Program	Enrollments as of October 15, 1997	Admissions Aug. 1, 1996 - July 31, 1997	Graduations Aug. 1, 1996 - July 31, 1997	Fall Admissions Aug. 1, 1997 - Dec. 31, 1997
	CALIFORNIA												
	- Continued												
081	Citrus College Mrs Marilyn Collins, Dept Chair *Chair's #: (626) 914-8721*	1000 W Foothill Blvd Glendora 91741				CC	PBL	12	12	24	156	46	52
020	City College of San Francisco Mrs Evelyn Massey Porter, Dir *Chair's #: (415) 561-1912*	1860 Hayes St San Francisco 94117				CC	PBL			Publication withheld			
745	Clovis Adult Sch & Voc Ed Mrs Lola L Gasperetti, Director *Chair's #: (209) 298-2172*	1452 David E Cook Way Clovis 92611				SEC	PBL			Publication withheld			
712	Coll of the Canyons Dr Kathleen Welch, Dir *Chair's #: (805) 259-7800 Ext 3366*	26455 N Rockwell Canyon Valencia 91355				CC	PBL			Publication withheld			
075	Coll of the Desert (2 Campuses) Mrs Celia Hartley, Chair *Chair's #: (760) 773-2580*	43-500 Monterey Ave Palm Desert 92260				CC	PBL	12	12	40	45	26	46
045	Coll of the Redwoods (3 Campuses) Ms Sandra Siddall, Dir *Chair's #: (707) 445-6770*	7351 Thompkins Hill Rd Eureka 95501				CC	PBL			55	58	0	60
708	Coll of the Siskiyous Mrs Gerri L Perry, Director *Chair's #: (530) 938-5270*	800 College Ave Weed 96094				CC	PBL			Publication withheld			
029	Compton College Ms Mary Montgomery, Dir *Chair's #: (310) 637-2660 Ext 2700*	1111 E Artesia Blvd Compton 90221				CC	PBL			Publication withheld			
044	Compton Unified Sch Dist Ms Lillian Giles, Dir *Chair's #: (310) 603-1829*	3663 Martin Luther King Blvd Lynwood 90262				GOV	PBL			Publication withheld			
098	Concorde Career Inst Ms Sybil Damon, Dir *Chair's #: (909) 884-8891 Ext 24*	570 W 4th St San Bernardino 92401				TCH	PVT			Publication withheld			
010	Concorde Career Inst Mrs Muriel Owen, Dir *Chair's #: (619) 688-0800 Ext 32*	123 Camino De La Reina San Diego 92108				TCH	PVT	12	12	26	34	26	10
085	Concorde Career Inst-Valley College Mrs Georgene Tacke, Dir *Chair's #: (818) 766-8151 Ext 252*	12412 Victory Blvd North Hollywood 95823				TCH	PVT	12	12	180	210	190	60
005	Concorde Career Institute Ms Carol A Falde, Dir *Chair's #: (714) 635-3450*	1717 South Brookhurst Anaheim 92840				TCH	PVT	12	12	178	270	120	90

School Code	Name of School, Director of Program, and Phone Number	Street Address / City or Town and Zip Code	Footnotes	Type of Program	NLNAC Accreditation as of January 31, 1998	Administrative Control	Financial Support (principal source)	Number of Months in Program	Educational Requirements for Entering Adult Program	Enrollments as of October 15, 1997	Admissions Aug. 1, 1996 - July 31, 1997	Graduations Aug. 1, 1996 - July 31, 1997	Fall Admissions Aug. 1, 1997 - Dec. 31, 1997
	CALIFORNIA												
	- Continued												
055	De Anza Comm Coll Mrs Georgeanne Adamay, Actiing Head *Chair's #: (408) 864-8775*	21250 Stevens Creek Blvd Cupertino 95014	7			TCH	PBL			Data reported w/AD prog			
035	Emanuel Turlock PN Prog Mrs Judith Black, Director *Chair's #: (209) 669-2305*	825 Delbon Ave Turlock 95380				TCH	PBL	18	12	29	30	29	0
067	Four D Success Academy Dr Cherry Houston, Dir *Chair's #: (909) 783-9331*	952 So Mt Vernon Suite B Calton 92324				TCH	PBL			Publication withheld			
094	Gavilan College Mrs Kay Bedell, Director *Chair's #: (408) 848-4883*	5055 Santa Teresa Blvd Gilroy 95020				CC	PBL	12	12	37	24	20	24
011	Glendale Career College Ms Jean Nix, Dir *Chair's #: (818) 243-1131 Ext 263*	1021 Grandview Ave Glendale 91201				TCH	PVT	14	12	197	180	39	45
030	Glendale College Dr Sharon Hall, Assoc Dean *Chair's #: (818) 240-1000 Ext 5673*	1500 N Verdugo Rd Glendale 91208				CC	PBL	12	12	39	47	34	24
749	Grant Adult & Comm Ed Mrs Maxine Times, Director *Chair's #: (916) 263-6511*	3701 Stephen Dr N Highlands 95660				TCH	PBL			Publication withheld			
046	Grossmont Hlth Occupations Center Mrs B Patricia Twyman, Director *Chair's #: (619) 579-4780*	9368 Oakbourne Rd Santee 92071				SEC	PBL	15	12	55	60	62	0
741	Hacienda-La Puente Adult Educ Mrs Elda Pichetto, Dir *Chair's #: (818) 855-3138*	15325 E Los Robles Hacienda Heights 91745				SEC	PBL			Publication withheld			
077	Hanford Adult School (2 Campuses) Mrs Karen Ormsby, Director *Chair's #: (209) 583-0856 Ext 60*	120 E Grangeville Blvd Hanford 93230				SEC	PBL			Publication withheld			
039	Hartnell College Mrs Colly Tettelbach, Dir *Chair's #: (408) 755-6771*	156 Homestead Ave Salinas 93901				CC	PBL			Publication withheld			
060	Imperial Valley College Dr Betty Marks, Admin *Chair's #: (619) 352-8320*	PO Box 158 Imperial 92251				CC	PBL			Publication withheld			
736	Lassen Comm College Ms Liona Maas, Dir *Chair's #: (916) 251-8870*	PO Box 3000 Susanville 96130				CC	PBL			Publication withheld			

Explanation of footnotes on page x

School Code	Name of School, Director of Program, and Phone Number	Street Address, City or Town and Zip Code	Footnotes	Type of Program	NLNAC Accreditation as of January 31, 1998	Administrative Control	Financial Support (principal source)	Number of Months in Program	Educational Requirements for Entering Adult Program	Enrollments as of October 15, 1997	Admissions Aug. 1, 1996 - July 31, 1997	Graduations Aug. 1, 1996 - July 31, 1997	Fall Admissions Aug. 1, 1997 - Dec. 31, 1997
071	Long Beach City College Mrs Verla Beck, Dir Chair's #: (562) 938-4166	4901 E Carson St Long Beach 90808				CC	PBL			Publication withheld			
013	Los Angeles Trade-Tech Coll-VN Prog Mrs Jo Ann Williams, Dir Chair's #: (213) 744-9453	400 W Washington Blvd Los Angeles 90015				CC	PBL			Publication withheld			
719	Los Angeles Unified Sch District Mrs Lillian Goodman, Director Chair's #: (213) 625-6649	1320 W 3rd St, Rm 216 Los Angeles 90017				TCH	PBL			90	105	95	90
027	Los Medanos College Ms Eva Murray, Director Chair's #: (925) 439-2181	2700 E Leland Rd Pittsburg 94565				CC	PBL			27	30	25	0
748	Lynwood Unified Sch Dist Mrs Elizabeth McCray, Dir Chair's #: (310) 604-1786	12124 Bullis Rd Lynwood 90262				SEC	PBL			Publication withheld			
072	Marian College Mrs Cirlezita Cabote, Dir Chair's #: (213) 388-3566	3325 Wishire Blvd Suite 1213 Los Angeles 90010	1			COL	PVT			Publication withheld			
739	Maric College (2 Campuses) Mrs Phyllis Crownover, Dir Chair's #: (619) 654-3604	3666 Kearny Villa Rd San Diego 92123				TCH	PVT			Publication withheld			
043	Merced College Ms Penny Sawyer, Dir Chair's #: (209) 384-6128	3600 M St Merced 95348	7			CC	PBL			Data reported w/AD prog			
003	Merritt College Mrs Carol A Lee, Director Chair's #: (510) 436-2506	12500 Campus Dr Oakland 94619	7			CC	PBL			Data reported w/AD prog			
073	Mira Costa College Ms Katherine M Herd, Director Chair's #: (760) 757-2121 Ext 6842	One Barnard Dr Oceanside 92056				CC	PBL	18		34	30	22	15
083	Mission College Dr Mary Moore, Chair Chair's #: (408) 748-2748	3000 Mission College Blvd Santa Clara 95054				CC	PBL	18	12	90	60	56	30
062	Mt San Jacinto College Mrs Judy Gentry, Dir Chair's #: (909) 672-6752 Ext 2609	28237 La Piedra Rd Menifee 92584				CC	PBL	18	12	52	36	21	24
015	Napa Valley College Ms Patty Vail, Dean Chair's #: (707) 253-3120	2277 Napa-Vallejo Hwy Napa 94558				CC	PBL	12	12	67	73	21	0

School Code	Name of School, Director of Program, and Phone Number	Street Address / City or Town and Zip Code		Footnotes	Type of Program	NLNAC Accreditation as of January 31, 1998	Administrative Control	Financial Support (principal source)	Number of Months in Program	Educational Requirements for Entering Adult Program	Enrollments as of October 15, 1997	Admissions Aug. 1, 1996 - July 31, 1997	Graduations Aug. 1, 1996 - July 31, 1997	Fall Admissions Aug. 1, 1997 - Dec. 31, 1997
	CALIFORNIA													
	- Continued													
746	North Orange County ROP Mrs Janine O' Buchon, Director *Chair's #: (714) 635-1281 Ext 14*	1617 E Ball Rd Anaheim	92805				TCH	PBL	13	12	60	120	85	60
099	Oxnard Adult Sch-Voc Prog Dr Dorothy Phillips, Coord *Chair's #: (805) 385-2578*	280 Skyway Dr Commarita	93010				SEC	PBL		Publication withheld				
058	Palo Verde Comm Coll Ms D Malishan Dumas, Assoc Dean *Chair's #: (760) 921-5344*	811 West Chansloway Blythe	92225				CC	PBL	15	12	15	16	11	15
001	Pasadena City College Ms Mary Wynn, Dean *Chair's #: (626) 585-7325*	1570 E Colorado Blvd Pasadena	91106		7		CC	PBL	14	12	23	35	24	37
705	Pittsburg Adult Ed Mrs Bridget P Teranen, Director *Chair's #: (510) 473-4467*	20 E 10th St Pittsburg	94565				TCH	PBL		Publication withheld				
750	Plumas & Sierra Counties ROP Mr Paul Mrowcznski, Director *Chair's #: (916) 283-6500 Ext 213*	PO Box P Quincy	95971				TCH	PBL		Publication withheld				
082	Porterville College Ms Valerie Lombardi, Dir *Chair's #: (209) 791-2322*	100 E College Ave Porterville	93257				CC	PBL		Publication withheld				
751	Poway Unified Sch Dist ROP Mrs Nancy A Allen, Director *Chair's #: (619) 679-0158*	12450 Glenoak Rd Poway	92064				SEC	PBL	15		23	0	17	23
735	Redlands Unified Sch Dist-Adult Sch Ms Pam Hinckley, Chair *Chair's #: (909) 307-5315 Ext 335*	7 West Delaware Ave Redlands	92373				SEC	PBL		Publication withheld				
063	Rio Hondo Jr College Mrs Marcia McCormick, Dir *Chair's #: (562) 692-0921 Ext 3596*	3600 Workman Mill Rd Whittier	90608				CC	PBL	10	12	48	48	37	48
017	Riverside Comm College Dr Donna Schutte, Interim Dir *Chair's #: (909) 222-8408*	4800 Magnolia Ave Riverside	92506				CC	PBL	12	12	84	61	47	58
033	Sacramento City College VN Prog Mrs Diane Welch, Dir *Chair's #: (916) 558-2275*	3835 Freeport Blvd Sacramento	95822				CC	PBL		Publication withheld				
066	San Bernardino Adult School Ms Pam Hinckley, Dir *Chair's #: (909) 388-6051*	1200 N "E" St San Bernardino	92405				TCH	PBL		Publication withheld				

Explanation of footnotes on page x

School Code	Name of School, Director of Program, and Phone Number	Street Address / City or Town and Zip Code		Footnotes	Type of Program	NLNAC Accreditation as of January 31, 1998	Administrative Control	Financial Support (principal source)	Number of Months in Program	Educational Requirements for Entering Adult Program	Enrollments as of October 15, 1997	Admissions Aug. 1, 1996 - July 31, 1997	Graduations Aug. 1, 1996 - July 31, 1997	Fall Admissions Aug. 1, 1997 - Dec. 31, 1997
	CALIFORNIA													
	- Continued													
036	San Joaquin Delta Comm College Mrs Virginia Antaran, Director *Chair's #: (209) 954-5516 Ext 5502*	5151 Pacific Ave Stockton	95207	7			CC	PBL	12	12	30	30	30	0
048	Santa Barbara City College Ms Jacqueline Huth, Director *Chair's #: (805) 964-7678 Ext 2233*	721 Cliff Dr Santa Barbara	93109				CC	PBL	18	12	19	25	0	0
042	Santa Rosa Jr College Ms Joan Scarborough, Director *Chair's #: (707) 527-4271 Ext 4529*	1501 Mendocino Dr Santa Rosa	95401				CC	PBL	18	12	26	31	30	0
026	Shasta College Ms Georgianne Dinkel, Director *Chair's #: (530) 225-4725*	11555 Old OR Trail Redding	96049				CC	PBL	18	12	29	30	30	0
054	Sierra College Ms Margaret White, Assoc Dean *Chair's #: (916) 781-0556*	5000 Rocklin Rd Rocklin	95677	7			CC	PBL			Data reported w/AD prog			
092	Simi Vly Adult Sch Mrs Lois Harrion, Dir *Chair's #: (805) 579-6260*	3192 Los Angeles Ave Simi Valley	93065				TCH	PBL	12	12	17	23	21	18
069	Southwestern College Ms Charlotte A Erdahl, Dean *Chair's #: (619) 482-6352*	900 Otay Lakes Rd Chula Vista	92010				CC	PBL	18	12	39	0	27	39
097	St Francis Career Coll Mrs Marilyn Overby, Dir *Chair's #: (310) 603-1830*	3630 E Imperial Highway Lynwood	90262		HSE		TCH TCH	PVT PVT	13 13	12 12	28 0	60 15	48 13	20 0
037	Summit Career College Ms Edda Coughran, Dir *Chair's #: (909) 422-8950*	1330 E Cooley Dr Colton	92324				TCH	PVT			89	34	112	34
079	Ukiah Adult Sch Voc Nsg Prog Mrs Ruby Rose, Director *Chair's #: (707) 463-5217*	1056 N Bush St Ukiah	95482				TCH	PBL	14	12	35	0	29	36
056	Western Career College Ms Debra Aucoin-Ratcliff, Dir *Chair's #: (916) 361-1660 Ext 714*	8909 Folson Blvd Sacramento	95826				TCH	PVT	18	12	47	44	33	47
040	Yuba College Ms Margot Loschke, Director *Chair's #: (916) 741-6785*	2088 N Beale Rd Marysville	95901				CC	PBL			Publication withheld			
078	YWCA Los Angeles Job Corps Ctr Miss Evangeline Malabanan, Dir *Chair's #: (213) 741-5316*	1106 S Broadway Los Angeles	90015				GOV	PBL			Publication withheld			

Explanation of footnotes on page x

School Code	Name of School, Director of Program, and Phone Number	Street Address / City or Town and Zip Code		Footnotes	Type of Program	NLNAC Accreditation as of January 31, 1998	Administrative Control	Financial Support (principal source)	Number of Months in Program	Educational Requirements for Entering Adult Program	Enrollments as of October 15, 1997	Admissions Aug. 1, 1996 - July 31, 1997	Graduations Aug. 1, 1996 - July 31, 1997	Fall Admissions Aug. 1, 1997 - Dec. 31, 1997
	COLORADO													
	17 Programs in 17 Schools													
006	Colorado Mt College Ms Susan Parker, Dir *Chair's #: (970) 945-7481*	3000 County Rd 114 Glenwood Spring	81601				CC	PBL			Publication withheld			
026	Comm College of Denver Mrs Vicki V Earnest, Coord *Chair's #: (303) 556-3842*	PO Box 173363 Denver	80217	7			CC	PBL			Data reported w/AD prog			
005	Concorde Career Institute Ms Jacqueline Verville, Dir *Chair's #: (303) 832-1690*	770 Grant St Denver	80203	1			TCH	PVT	13	12	87	115	83	37
021	Delta Montrose Area Voc Tech Sch Mrs Shari Barclay, Coord *Chair's #: (970) 874-7671 Ext 121*	1765 US Hwy 50 Delta	81416				TCH	PBL	10	12	35	27	21	26
002	Emily Griffith Opportunity School Dr E Ford-Pade, Dir *Chair's #: (303) 575-4737*	1250 Welton St Lakewood	80226				TCH	PBL			Publication withheld			
017	FRCC/Larimer County Center Ms Audrey Bopp, Coord *Chair's #: (970) 226-1119 Ext 203*	4616 S Shields Fort Collins	80526	7			CC	PBL			Data reported w/AD prog			
013	Front Range Comm Coll Mrs Merrilee McDuffie, Dir *Chair's #: (303) 516-8001*	5490 Spine Rd Boulder	80301				CC	PBL	9	12	41	38	32	36
029	Front Range Comm College Mrs Alma L Mueller, Dir *Chair's #: (303) 404-5204*	3645 W 112th Ave Westminster	80030	7			CC	PBL			Data reported w/AD prog			
010	Lamar Comm College Mrs Sandy Summers, Dir *Chair's #: (719) 336-2248 Ext 415*	2401 South Main St Lamar	81052				TCH	PBL	11	12	20	25	20	21
015	Northeastern Jr College, PN Prog Mrs Betty Brunner, Coordinator *Chair's #: (970) 522-6600 Ext 6749*	100 College St Sterling	80751				CC	PBL	11	12	28	16	16	17
028	Otero Jr College Mrs Denise Root, Dir *Chair's #: (719) 384-6894*	La Junta	81050	7			CC	PBL			Data reported w/AD prog			
009	Pueblo Comm College (2 Branches) Mrs Dora Hallock, Chair *Chair's #: (719) 549-3409 Ext 3279*	900 W Orman Pueblo	81004			A	TCH	PBL	9	12	64	66	43	63
027	San Juan Basin Tech Sch Mrs Nancy Brown, Dir *Chair's #: (970) 565-8457 Ext 129*	Po Box 970 Cortez	81321		HSE		TCH TCH	PBL PBL	10 9	12 12	27 0	31 0	28 0	28 0

Explanation of footnotes on page x

School Code	Name of School, Director of Program, and Phone Number	Street Address / City or Town and Zip Code		Footnotes	Type of Program	NLNAC Accreditation as of January 31, 1998	Administrative Control	Financial Support (principal source)	Number of Months in Program	Educational Requirements for Entering Adult Program	Enrollments as of October 15, 1997	Admissions Aug. 1, 1996 - July 31, 1997	Graduations Aug. 1, 1996 - July 31, 1997	Fall Admissions Aug. 1, 1997 - Dec. 31, 1997
	COLORADO													
	- Continued													
016	T H Pickens Ctr/Aurora Public Schs Ms Candace Pritchard, Instructor *Chair's #: (303) 344-4910*	500 Buckley Rd Aurora	80011				TCH	PBL			Publication withheld			
008	Trinidad State Jr College Sch of PN Ms Judie E Stickel, Director *Chair's #: (719) 846-5524*	600 Prospect St Trinidad	81082				CC	PBL			Publication withheld			
	CONNECTICUT													
	12 Programs in 12 Schools													
053	A I Prince Voc Techs Sch Mrs Gayle Whitmore, Dept Head *Chair's #: (860) 566-1867*	500 Brookfield St Hartford	06106				TCH	PBL	0		29	41	29	0
050	Bullard Havens Reg Voc-Tech Sch Miss Rita M Lambert, Dept Head *Chair's #: (203) 579-6117*	500 Palisades Ave Bridgeport	06610				TCH	PBL	15	12	43	50	37	0
051	E C Goodwin Reg Voc-Tech Sch Mrs Maureen Rabito, Dept Head *Chair's #: (860) 827-7731*	735 Slater Rd New Britain	06053				TCH	PBL	14	12	40	40	28	40
055	Eli Whitney Reg Voc-Tech Sch Mrs Joan T Novarro, Dept Head *Chair's #: (203) 397-4035*	71 Jones Rd Hamden	06514				TCH	PBL	14	12	31	42	27	0
058	Henry Abbott Reg Voc-Tech Sch Mrs Pamela P Cramer, Dept Head *Chair's #: (203) 797-2724*	Hayestown Rd Danbury	06810				TCH	PVT	13	12	32	45	32	0
052	Howell Cheney Voc-Tech Sch Ms Barbara Lindner, Dept Head *Chair's #: (860) 253-3191*	791 W Middle Tpke Manchester	06040				TCH	PBL			Publication withheld			
010	J M Wright Reg Voc-Tech Sch Mrs Maureen Wright Maher, Head *Chair's #: (203) 324-7363 Ext 33*	Scalzi Pk Stamford	06904				SEC	PBL	12	12	21	34	20	0
057	Kaynor Reg Voc-Tech Sch Mrs Judy Leonardi, Dept Head *Chair's #: (203) 596-4302 Ext 33*	43 Tomkins St Waterbury	06708				TCH	PBL	13	12	40	40	40	40
023	Morse Sch Business Miss Eleanor Davio, Manager *Chair's #: (860) 522-2261 Ext 148*	275 Asylum St Hartford	06904				TCH	PVT			Publication withheld			
011	Norwich Reg Voc-Tech Sch Mrs Karen McKenney, Head *Chair's #: (860) 886-5669*	590 New London Tpke Norwich	06360				TCH	PBL	15	12	34	40	39	0

Explanation of footnotes on page x

School Code	Name of School, Director of Program, and Phone Number	Street Address / City or Town and Zip Code		Footnotes	Type of Program	NLNAC Accreditation as of January 31, 1998	Administrative Control	Financial Support (principal source)	Number of Months in Program	Educational Requirements for Entering Adult Program	Enrollments as of October 15, 1997	Admissions Aug. 1, 1996 - July 31, 1997	Graduations Aug. 1, 1996 - July 31, 1997	Fall Admissions Aug. 1, 1997 - Dec. 31, 1997
	CONNECTICUT													
	- Continued													
059	Vinal Reg Voc-Tech Sch / Mrs Margaret Andrews, Dept Head / *Chair's #: (860) 344-7141*	60 Daniels St / Middletown	06457				TCH	PBL	15	12	24	30	28	30
056	Windham Reg Voc-Tech Sch / Ms Maryann Donovan, Dept Head / *Chair's #: (860) 456-3879 Ext 156*	210 Birch St / Willimantic	06226				TCH	PBL			Publication withheld			
	DELAWARE													
	4 Programs in 3 Schools													
005	DE Tech & Comm College-Southern Ca / Mrs Judith Caldwell, Chair / *Chair's #: (302) 855-1614*	PO Box 610 / Georgetown	19947				CC	PBL	11	12	24	25	19	24
004	DE Tech & Comm College-Terry Camp / Ms Ruth Yanos, Chair / *Chair's #: (302) 739-5444*	1832 N Dupont Pkwy / Dover	19901				CC	PBL	12	12	29	31	26	29
012	Delcastle Voc-Tech HS / Mrs Janet West, Director / *Chair's #: (302) 995-5619*	1417 Newport Rd / Wilmington	19804				TCH	PBL			Publication withheld			
	DISTRICT OF COLUMBIA													
	3 Programs in 3 Schools													
004	Harrison Center For Career Educ / Mrs Arthuretta Zeigler, Dir / *Chair's #: (202) 628-5672 Ext 308*	624 9th St NW / Washington	20007			A	IND	PVT	12	12	57	53	60	28
005	Health Management Inc / Ms Eleanor Browning, Exec Dir / *Chair's #: (202) 291-9020*	6856 Eastern Ave NW 376 / Washington	20012				IND	PVT			Publication withheld			
003	Margaret Murray Washington Voc HS / Dr Ruth Richardson, Coord / *Chair's #: (202) 673-7436 Ext 202*	27 O St NW / Washington	20001		HSE	A / A	TCH / TCH	PBL / PBL			Publication withheld			
	FLORIDA													
	44 Programs in 44 Schools													
013	Academy For Practical Nursing / Mrs Lois Gackenheimer, Dir / *Chair's #: (561) 683-1400*	5154 Okeechobee Blvd Suite 2 / West Palm Beach	33417		2		SEC	PVT	12	12	45	47	0	0
002	Allied Hlth Training Center Inc / Ms Beverly Pryce, Dir / *Chair's #: (954) 961-9466*	4350 W Hallandale / Hollywood	33023				TCH	PVT			Publication withheld			
038	Brevard Comm College / Mrs Jene M Holland, Chair / *Chair's #: (407) 632-1111*	1519 Clearlake Rd / Cocoa	32922				CC	PBL	12	12	21	24	24	0

Explanation of footnotes on page x

School Code	Name of School, Director of Program, and Phone Number	Street Address / City or Town and Zip Code	Footnotes	Type of Program	NLNAC Accreditation as of January 31, 1998	Administrative Control	Financial Support (principal source)	Number of Months in Program	Educational Requirements for Entering Adult Program	Enrollments as of October 15, 1997	Admissions Aug. 1, 1996 - July 31, 1997	Graduations Aug. 1, 1996 - July 31, 1997	Fall Admissions Aug. 1, 1997 - Dec. 31, 1997
	FLORIDA - Continued												
024	Broward Co Pract Nsg Progs (4 Centers) Ms Barbara L Zygowsky, Specialist *Chair's #: (954) 760-7409*	600 SE 3rd Ave Fort Lauderdale 33301			A	TCH	PBL			Publication withheld			
053	Central Florida Comm College Dr Gwen Lapham-Alcorn, Assoc Dean *Chair's #: (352) 237-2111 Ext 275*	3001 SW College Rd Ocala 32674			A	CC	PBL	12	12	29	36	26	0
044	Charlotte Co Voc-Tech Ctr Mrs Yvonne B Meinket, Supervisor *Chair's #: (941) 629-6819 Ext 136*	18300 Toledo Blade Blvd Port Charlotte 33948				TCH	PBL			Publication withheld			
022	Chipola Jr College Mrs Kathy Wheeler, Dir *Chair's #: (850) 718-2278 Ext 2278*	3094 Indian Circle Marianna 32466	7			CC	PBL	12	12	24	24	19	0
007	Dade Co Public Schs (4 Centers) Ms Rose Hodge, Chair *Chair's #: (305) 995-2827*	1450 NE 2nd Ave Rm 816 Miami 33132			A	TCH	PBL			Publication withheld			
020	Daytona Beach Comm College Ms Barbara Doyle, Chair *Chair's #: (904) 255-8131 Ext 3720*	1200 Volusia Ave Box 2811 Daytona Beach 32120				CC	PBL	11	12	36	96	51	37
047	Desoto County PN Prog Ms Janet Loporto, Instructor *Chair's #: (941) 494-4222 Ext 148*	530 La Solono Ave Arcadia 33821				SEC	PBL	11	12	12	12	11	12
031	Florida Comm College at Jacksonville Mrs Donna Perry, Chair *Chair's #: (904) 766-6550*	4501 Capper Rd Campus C212 Jacksonville 32218				CC	PBL			Publication withheld			
026	Florida Hosp College of Hlth Sciences Mrs Cheryl Galusha, Chair *Chair's #: (407) 895-7893*	795 Lake Estelle Dr Orlando 32803				CC	PVT	11	12	37	30	22	40
015	Gadsden Tech Inst Ms Glenda Battle, Coord *Chair's #: (850) 875-8324 Ext 129*	201 Martin Luther King Blvd Quincy 32351	2			TCH	PBL			Publication withheld			
006	Hillsborough Co-Erwin V-T Ctr Mrs Cheryl Brown, Dept Head *Chair's #: (813) 231-1800 Ext 2447*	2010 E Hillsborough Ave Tampa 33610				TCH	PBL	12	12	153	233	149	59
004	Hlth Inst of Tampa Bay Ms Sharon A Roberts, Dir *Chair's #: (813) 577-1497*	9549 Koger Blvd Suite 100 St Petersburg 33702				IND	PVT			131	144	98	61
033	Indian River Comm College Ms Jane P Cebelak, Director *Chair's #: (561) 462-4778*	3209 Virginia Ave Fort Pierce 34981				CC	PBL	11	11	77	58	63	0

FLORIDA

- Continued

School Code	Name of School, Director of Program, and Phone Number	Street Address, City or Town and Zip Code	Footnotes	Type of Program	NLNAC Accreditation as of January 31, 1998	Administrative Control	Financial Support (principal source)	Number of Months in Program	Educational Requirements for Entering Adult Program	Enrollments as of October 15, 1997	Admissions Aug. 1, 1996 - July 31, 1997	Graduations Aug. 1, 1996 - July 31, 1997	Fall Admissions Aug. 1, 1997 - Dec. 31, 1997
035	James L Walker Tech Ctr Mrs Sally Holland, Coord Chair's #: (941) 643-0919 Ext 6655	3702 Estey Ave, N Naples 34104				TCH	PBL	12	12	67	72	60	48
057	Lake City Comm College Mrs Judy Clemons, Coord Chair's #: (904) 752-1822 Ext 1155	Route 19 Box 1030 Lake City 32025				CC	PBL	12	12	21	24	26	0
032	Lake County Area Voc-Tech Ctr Ms Elaine Rejimbal, Chair Chair's #: (352) 742-6497	2001 Kurt St Eustis 32726				TCH	PBL	11	12	53	60	40	31
029	Lee County Sch of PN Mrs Sheila Sarver, Dir Chair's #: (941) 334-4544 Ext 342	3800 Michigan Ave Fort Myers 33916				TCH	PBL			Publication withheld			
011	Lively Tech Ctr Ms Judith G Hankin, Dir Chair's #: (904) 487-7452	500 N Appleyard Dr Tallahassee 32304				TCH	PBL			Publication withheld			
027	Manatee Tech Inst Mrs Faith Herring, Chair Chair's #: (941) 751-7957	5603 34th St West Bradenton 34210				TCH	PBL	12	12	56	70	54	35
045	Mercy Hospital Mr James Bray, Dir Chair's #: (305) 285-2777 Ext 2544	3663 S Miami Ave Miami 33133			A	HSP	PVT			Publication withheld			
021	North Florida Comm Coll Mr Karen Steward, Dir Chair's #: (904) 973-2288 Ext 134	1000 Turner Davis Dr Madison 32340				CC	PBL			Publication withheld			
005	Oklaloosa Applied Tech Center Mrs Sylvia Austin, Dept Head Chair's #: (904)-833-3500 Ext 3544	1976 Lewis Turner Blvd Ft Walton Beach 32547				TCH	PBL			Publication withheld			
023	OrangeTech Ed Ctr-Orlando Tech Mrs Yvonne Julien, Chair Chair's #: (407) 317-3371	301 W Amelia St Orlando 32801				TCH	PBL	12	12	109	142	95	50
025	Palm Beach Co PN Program (3 Centers) Mrs Donna Jordan, Specialist Chair's #: (561) 434-7467	3312 Forest Hill Blvd #A330 West Palm Beach 33406				TCH	PBL	0	12	139	133	60	67
046	Pasco-Hernando Comm College Ms Karen Richardson, Dir Chair's #: (813) 847-2727 Ext 3280	10230 Ridge Rd New Port Richey 34654				CC	PBL	10	11	72	72	41	48
003	Pensacola Jr College Dr Joan Connell, Dept Head Chair's #: (850) 484-2254	5555 W Hwy 98 Pensacola 32507				CC	PBL	12		82	94	43	0

School Code	Name of School, Director of Program, and Phone Number	Street Address / City or Town and Zip Code	Footnotes	Type of Program	NLNAC Accreditation as of January 31, 1998	Administrative Control	Financial Support (principal source)	Number of Months in Program	Educational Requirements for Entering Adult Program	Enrollments as of October 15, 1997	Admissions Aug. 1, 1996 - July 31, 1997	Graduations Aug. 1, 1996 - July 31, 1997	Fall Admissions Aug. 1, 1997 - Dec. 31, 1997
	FLORIDA												
	- Continued												
009	Pinellas Tech Educ Center Mrs Evelyn Gardner, Chair *Chair's #: (813) 893-2500 Ext 1071*	901 34th St, S St Petersburg 33711				TCH	PBL	12	12	101	96	86	180
016	Pinellas Tech Educ Ctr Mrs Candace Gioia, Chair *Chair's #: (813) 538-7167 Ext 1128*	6100 154th Ave, N Clearwater 34620				TCH	PBL	12	11	125	139	58	34
059	Port St Lucie Sch of PN Ms Mabel Smith-Duffus, Dir *Chair's #: (561) 398-0102*	10792 South Federal Highway Port St Lucie 34952				TCH	PBL	12	12	15	24	14	0
014	Santa Fe Comm College Ms Rita Sutherland, Dir *Chair's #: (352) 395-5703*	3000 NW 83rd St Box 1530 Gainesville 32606			A	CC	PBL	10	12	30	36	36	30
017	Sarasota Co Vocational Tech Inst Dr Linda Swisher, Chair *Chair's #: (941) 924-1365 Ext 372*	4748 Beneva Rd Sarasota 34233			A	TCH	PBL	12	12	56	40	52	40
030	Seminole Comm College Ms Sharon Cannon, Manager *Chair's #: (407) 328-2018*	100 Weldon Blvd Sanford 32773				CC	PBL	0		53	55	43	56
042	South Florida Comm College Dr Mary Ann Fritz, Chair *Chair's #: (941) 453-6661 Ext 118*	600 W College Dr Avon Park 33825				CC	PBL	11	12	21	24	45	23
028	St Augustine Tech Ctr Mrs Nancy Lee Thomas, Manager *Chair's #: (904) 829-1085 Ext 1085*	2980 Collins Avenue St Augustine 32095				TCH	PBL	12	12	46	48	46	24
037	Suwannee-Hamilton Area Vo-Tech Ctr Mrs Virginia Stebbins, Director *Chair's #: (904) 364-2784 Ext 2784*	415 SW Pinewood Dr Live Oak 32060				TCH	PBL	11	12	17	17	19	19
061	Technical Education Center Ms Karen Guritz, Director *Chair's #: (407) 344-5080 Ext 128*	501 Simpson Rd Kissimmee 34744				TCH	PBL			Publication withheld			
019	Tom P Haney Tech Center Ms Lanita Hill, Director *Chair's #: (904) 769-2191 Ext 111*	3016 Hwy 77 Panama City 32405				TCH	PBL			Publication withheld			
010	Traviss Tech Center Ms JoAnn Hagghloom, Dir *Chair's #: (941) 499-2700 Ext 2715*	3225 Winter Lake Rd Lakeland 33803				TCH	PBL			94	96	84	95
039	Washington-Holmes Tech Center Mrs Gena Porter-Lankist, Coord *Chair's #: (850) 638-1180 Ext 351*	209 Hoyt St Chipley 32428				TCH	PBL	11	12	38	44	29	14

School Code	Name of School, Director of Program, and Phone Number	Street Address City or Town and Zip Code		Footnotes	Type of Program	NLNAC Accreditation as of January 31, 1998	Administrative Control	Financial Support (principal source)	Number of Months in Program	Educational Requirements for Entering Adult Program	Enrollments as of October 15, 1997	Admissions Aug. 1, 1996 - July 31, 1997	Graduations Aug. 1, 1996 - July 31, 1997	Fall Admissions Aug. 1, 1997 - Dec. 31, 1997
	FLORIDA													
	- Continued													
043	Withlacoochee Tech Inst Mrs Jan Lesight, Coord *Chair's #: (352) 726-2430 Ext 233*	1201 W Main St Inverness	34450				TCH	PBL	10	12	22	24	22	12
	GEORGIA													
	48 Programs in 43 Schools													
019	Albany Tech Institute Mrs Dorothy K Garner, Dir *Chair's #: (912) 430-3061*	1021 Lowe Rd Albany	31708				TCH	PBL	15	12	69	111	34	36
011	Altamaha Tech Inst Dr C Paul Scott, President *Chair's #: (912) 427-5803*	1777 W Cherry St Jesup	31545				TCH	PBL		Publication withheld				
026	Athens Area Tech Inst Mrs Fay Joyce Manus, Dir *Chair's #: (706) 355-5058*	US Hwy 29 N Athens	30610				TCH	PBL		Publication withheld				
013	Atlanta Tech Inst Ms Patricia Blake, Chair *Chair's #: (404) 756-3719*	1560 Metropolitan Pkwy Atlanta	30310				TCH	PBL		Publication withheld				
050	Augusta Tech Institute (2 Divs) Mrs Sara Youngblood, Dept Head *Chair's #: (706) 771-4190*	3116 Deans Bridge Rd Augusta	30906			A	TCH	PBL	15	12	118	106	84	45
020	Bainbridge College Dr Robert U Coker, Chair *Chair's #: (912) 248-2530*	2500 E Shotwell St Bainbridge	31717				CC	PBL	15	12	31	21	11	20
032	Carroll Tech Inst Mrs Jane Parkman, Chair *Chair's #: (770) 836-6800*	997 So Hwy-16 Carrollton	30116	2			TCH	PBL		Publication withheld				
038	Chattahoochee Tech Institute (2 Divs) Mrs Marilyn Mintz, Lead Instructor *Chair's #: (770) 528-4568*	980 S Cobb Dr SE Marietta	30060				TCH	PBL	15	12	58	60	31	60
036	Coastal Ga Comm Coll Mrs Julia C Dent, Asst Prof *Chair's #: (912) 262-3340*	3700 Altama Ave Brunswick	31522				CC	PBL		Publication withheld				
074	Columbus Tech Institute Dr Margaret Gursel, Head *Chair's #: (706) 649-1800*	928 45th St Columbus	31904				TCH	PBL		Publication withheld				
007	Coosa Valley Tech Institute Dr Dorothy Gregg, Dir *Chair's #: (706) 295-6953*	785 Cedar Ave Rome	30161				TCH	PBL	15	12	60	60	27	30

Explanation of footnotes on page x

School Code	Name of School, Director of Program, and Phone Number	Street Address / City or Town and Zip Code	Footnotes	Type of Program	NLNAC Accreditation as of January 31, 1998	Administrative Control	Financial Support (principal source)	Number of Months in Program	Educational Requirements for Entering Adult Program	Enrollments as of October 15, 1997	Admissions Aug. 1, 1996 - July 31, 1997	Graduations Aug. 1, 1996 - July 31, 1997	Fall Admissions Aug. 1, 1997 - Dec. 31, 1997
	GEORGIA - Continued												
024	Dalton Coll-PN Prog Mrs Carolyn Higgins, Coord *Chair's #: (706) 278-8922*	1221 Elkwood Dr Dalton 30720				TCH	PBL	15	12	39	53	22	33
037	DeKalb Tech Institute Ms Geri Moreland, Dept Chair *Chair's #: (404) 297-9522 Ext 128*	495 N Indian Creek Dr Clarkston 30021				TCH	PBL			Publication withheld			
072	East Central Tech Institute (2 Divs) Dr Diane Harper, President *Chair's #: (912) 468-7487 Ext 2108*	PO Box 1069 667 Perry House Fitzgerald 31750				TCH	PBL			Publication withheld			
040	Flint River Tech Inst (2 Divs) Mrs F McDowell, Lead Instructor *Chair's #: (706) 646-6185 Ext 6181*	Box 1089 US Hwy 19 South Thomaston 30286				TCH	PBL			Publication withheld			
017	Griffin Technical Inst Ms Joyce Hickey, Dept Head *Chair's #: (770) 228-7348*	501 Varsity Rd Griffin 30223				TCH	PBL			Publication withheld			
091	Gwinnett Tech Inst Ms Drinda Taylor, Dir *Chair's #: (404) 962-7580 Ext 178*	5150 Sugarloaf Parkway Lawrenceville 30246				TCH	PBL			Publication withheld			
097	Heart of GA Tech Inst (2 Branches) Mrs June Williams, Chair *Chair's #: (912) 374-7122*	560 Pinehill Rd Dublin 31021				TCH	PBL			Publication withheld			
084	Lanier Tech Institute Mrs Gail Adam, Instructor *Chair's #: (404) 531-6300 Ext 6371*	PO Box 58 2990 Landrum Edu Oakwood 30566				TCH	PBL			Publication withheld			
043	Macon Tech Baldwin, County Ms Sue Hodell, Dept Chair *Chair's #: (912) 445-1716*	PO Box 1009 Hwy 49 W Milledgeville 31061				TCH	PBL			Publication withheld			
009	Macon Tech Institute (2 Divs) Mrs Teresa Wilkins, Dept Head *Chair's #: (912) 757-3585*	3300 Macon Tech Dr Macon 31206				TCH	PBL	15	12	290	171	87	45
083	Middle GA Tech Institute Ms Julia Nell Shaw, Director *Chair's #: (912) 929-6800 Ext 130*	1311 Corder Rd Warner Robins 31088				TCH	PBL			Publication withheld			
066	Moultrie Area Tech Inst (2 Divs) Earlene Sizemore, Vice President *Chair's #: (912) 891-7000*	361 Industrial Dr Moultrie 31768				TCH	PBL			Publication withheld			
015	North Georgia Tech Inst (2 Branches) Mrs Melinda Shiflet, Instructor *Chair's #: (706) 754-7762*	GA Hwy 197 N Po Box 65 Clarkesville 30523				TCH	PBL			Publication withheld			

School Code	Name of School, Director of Program, and Phone Number	Street Address / City or Town and Zip Code	Footnotes	Type of Program	NLNAC Accreditation as of January 31, 1998	Administrative Control	Financial Support (principal source)	Number of Months in Program	Educational Requirements for Entering Adult Program	Enrollments as of October 15, 1997	Admissions Aug. 1, 1996 - July 31, 1997	Graduations Aug. 1, 1996 - July 31, 1997	Fall Admissions Aug. 1, 1997 - Dec. 31, 1997
	GEORGIA **- Continued**												
903	Ogeechee Tech Inst Mrs Carol Turknett, Instructor *Chair's #: (912) 871-1627*	One Joe Kennedy Blvd Statesboro 30458				TCH	PBL	18	12	73	17	19	13
010	Okefenokee Tech Inst Ms Willene Griffin Fox, Dir *Chair's #: (912) 287-6584 Ext 5836*	1701 Carswell Ave Waycross 31503				TCH	PBL	Publication withheld					
065	Pickens Tech Inst Ms Nancy Proffitt, Pres *Chair's #: (706) 692-4500*	100 Pickens Tech Dr Jasper 30143				TCH	PBL	15	12	60	48	42	24
063	Putnam Co School PN Mrs Cheryl Kimbrell, Instructor *Chair's #: (706) 485-2711 Ext 344*	101 Lake Oconee Pwy Box 43 Eatonton 31024				HSP	PBL	12		5	6	6	6
001	Sauderville Reg Tech Inst Ms Leslie Thigpen ; Coord *Chair's #: ((912) 553-2050*	1189 Deepsted Rd Box 61794 Sandersville 31082	2			TCH	PBL	Publication withheld					
008	Savannah Tech Sch (2 Branches) Mrs Victoria Agyekum, Dir *Chair's #: (912) 351-4554*	5717 White Bluff Rd Savannah 31499			A	TCH	PBL	Publication withheld					
002	South Georgia Tech Inst (2 Branches) Mrs Joyce Dunmon, Chair *Chair's #: (912) 931-2447*	1583 Southerfield Rd Americus 31709				TCH	PBL	Publication withheld					
901	Southeastern Tech Inst (2 Branches) Mrs Linda Grancen, Instructor *Chair's #: (912) 537-0386 Ext 3002*	3001 E First St Vidalia 30474				TCH	PBL	Publication withheld					
039	Swainsboro Tech Inst Dr Richard Thornton, Vice Pres *Chair's #: (912) 237-6465*	346 Kite Rd Swainsboro 30401				TCH	PBL	Publication withheld					
041	Thomas Tech Inst Dr Annie McElroy, Dept Head *Chair's #: (912) 225-5200*	15689 US Hwy 19 N Thomasville 31792		HSE		TCH TCH	PBL PBL	18 18	12 12	50 0	60 0	19 0	0 0
052	Tift Sch of PN (Div of Moultrie) Ms Wanda Golden, Dir *Chair's #: (912) 382-2767*	302 E 14th St Tifton 31794				TCH	PBL	Publication withheld					
022	Valdosta Tech Inst Mrs Jackie Serrell, Chair *Chair's #: (912) 333-2110*	4089 Val -Tech Rd Box 928 Valdosta 31602				TCH	PBL	Publication withheld					
090	Walker Tech Institute Mrs Pat Caldwell, Coord *Chair's #: (706) 764-3718*	265 Bicentennial Trail Rock Spring 30739				TCH	PBL	15	12	44	75	31	25

Explanation of footnotes on page x

School Code	Name of School, Director of Program, and Phone Number	Street Address / City or Town and Zip Code	Footnotes	Type of Program	NLNAC Accreditation as of January 31, 1998	Administrative Control	Financial Support (principal source)	Number of Months in Program	Educational Requirements for Entering Adult Program	Enrollments as of October 15, 1997	Admissions Aug. 1, 1996 - July 31, 1997	Graduations Aug. 1, 1996 - July 31, 1997	Fall Admissions Aug. 1, 1997 - Dec. 31, 1997
	GEORGIA												
	- Continued												
012	West Georgia Tech Inst Ms Beverly Cochran, Dir *Chair's #: (706) 845-4323 Ext 5729*	303 Fort Dr La Grange 30240				TCH	PBL			Publication withheld			
	HAWAII												
	4 Programs in 4 Schools												
002	Hawaii Comm College Dr Elizabeth Ojala, Dir *Chair's #: (808) 974-7560*	Hilo 96720				CC	PBL			29	30	29	19
001	Kapiolani Comm College-Nursing Dept Mrs Joan Matsukawa, Chair *Chair's #: (807) 734-9301*	4303 Diamond Head Rd Honolulu 96814				CC	PBL	11	12	60	60	42	60
004	Kauai Comm College Mr Richard Carmichael, Dir *Chair's #: (808) 245-8255*	3-1901 Kaumualii Hwy Lihue Kauai 96766				CC	PBL	11	12	18	23	25	18
005	Maui Comm College-Career Ladder Mrs Nancy Johnson, Chair *Chair's #: (808) 984-3250*	310 Kaahumanu Ave Kahului Maui 96732	7			CC	PBL	11		65	41	57	0
	IDAHO												
	5 Programs in 5 Schools												
026	Boise State Univ-Dept of Nsg Dr Anne Payne, Assoc Dean *Chair's #: (208) 385-3845*	1910 Univ Dr Boise 83725				CC	PBL	11	12	34	50	39	20
024	Coll of SO Idaho Voc-Tech Sch Dr Claudeen R Buettner, Chair *Chair's #: (208) 733-9554 Ext 2155*	PO Box 1238 Twin Falls 83303				CC	PBL	11	12	30	30	28	20
046	Eastern Idaho Tech College Ms Rebecca Nelson, Coord *Chair's #: (208) 524-3000 Ext 3446*	1600 S 2500 E Idaho Falls 83404		HSE		TCH TCH	PBL PBL	15	12 12	32 0	39 1	0 0	0 0
030	Idaho State Univ Voc-Tech Sch Ms Prescilla LaHann, Coord *Chair's #: (208) 236-2507 Ext 2507*	741 SO 7th Box 8380 Pocatello 83209		HSE		TCH TCH	PBL PBL			35 0	44 0	35 0	0 0
043	North Idaho College Voc-Tech Sch Ms Joan Brogan, Dir *Chair's #: (208) 769-3480*	W 1000 Garden Ave Coeur D'Alene 83814	7			TCH	PBL	11	12	12	10	7	12
	ILLINOIS												
	41 Programs in 38 Schools												
056	Beck Area Voc Ctr Ms Janice Augustine, Director *Chair's #: (618) 473-2222*	6137 Beck Rd Red Bud 62278				SEC	PBL	11	12	39	66	53	26

School Code	Name of School, Director of Program, and Phone Number	Street Address / City or Town and Zip Code		Footnotes	Type of Program	NLNAC Accreditation as of January 31, 1998	Administrative Control	Financial Support (principal source)	Number of Months in Program	Educational Requirements for Entering Adult Program	Enrollments as of October 15, 1997	Admissions Aug. 1, 1996 - July 31, 1997	Graduations Aug. 1, 1996 - July 31, 1997	Fall Admissions Aug. 1, 1997 - Dec. 31, 1997
	ILLINOIS													
	- Continued													
028	Black Hawk College Dr Sally Flesch, Chair *Chair's #: (309) 796-1311 Ext 3319*	6600 34th Ave Moline	61265				CC	PBL	9	12	41	59	48	41
052	Capital Area Sch of PN Ms Jamie Hamilton, Coord *Chair's #: (217) 585-2160*	2201 Toronto Rd Springfield	62707			A	TCH	PBL			Publication withheld			
029	Carl Sandburg College Ms Alice Enderlin, Coord *Chair's #: (309) 341-5253*	2232 S Lake Storey Rd Galesburg	61401				CC	PBL			Publication withheld			
011	Chicago Public Schools Ms Sandra Webb, Coord *Chair's #: (773) 534-7890*	2045 W Jackson Chicago	60612			A	SEC	PBL			Publication withheld			
034	City College of Chi-Hlth Occup Careers Mrs M Ward-Ellison, Dir *Chair's #: (773) 451-2000 Ext 2016*	3901 S State Chicago	60609				TCH	PBL			Publication withheld			
001	City Colleges of Chicago-W Wright Coll Ms Ingrid Forsberg, Dir *Chair's #: (773) 489-8915*	1645 N California Chicago	60647				CC	PBL			Publication withheld			
025	Danville Area Comm College Mrs Ann Wagle, Dir *Chair's #: (217) 443-8814*	2000 E Main St Danville	61832				CC	PBL			Publication withheld			
004	Decatur School of PN-Area Voc Ctr Mrs Mary L Cookson, Dir *Chair's #: (217) 424-3075*	300 E Eldorado St Decatur	62523				TCH	PBL	12	12	44	41	30	30
057	Elgin Comm College Mrs Maryann Vaca, Assoc Dean *Chair's #: (847)888-7350*	1700 Spartan Dr Elgin	60123		7		CC	PBL			Data reported w/AD Prog			
003	F W Olin Voc School-Alton PN Prog Mrs Joann Peuterbaugh, Coord *Chair's #: (618) 463-2092*	4200 Humbert Rd Alton	62002				TCH	PBL	11	12	27	36	20	9
060	Heartland Comm College Ms Jacqueline Perley, Dir *Chair's #: (309) 827-0500 Ext 448*	1226 Towanda Ave Bloomington	61701		7		CC	PBL			Data reported w/AD Prog			
049	Highland Comm College Mrs Alice Nied, Dir *Chair's #: (815) 235-6121 Ext 315*	2998 Pearl City Rd Freeport	61032				CC	PBL			Publication withheld			
053	IL Eastern Comm Colleges Dist 529 Dr Judy Johnson, Assoc Dean *Chair's #: (618) 395-7777 Ext 2136*	305 North West St Olney	62450				CC	PBL	11	12	136	147	110	147

Explanation of footnotes on page x

School Code	Name of School, Director of Program, and Phone Number	Street Address / City or Town and Zip Code		Footnotes	Type of Program	NLNAC Accreditation as of January 31, 1998	Administrative Control	Financial Support (principal source)	Number of Months in Program	Educational Requirements for Entering Adult Program	Enrollments as of October 15, 1997	Admissions Aug. 1, 1996 - July 31, 1997	Graduations Aug. 1, 1996 - July 31, 1997	Fall Admissions Aug. 1, 1997 - Dec. 31, 1997
	ILLINOIS													
	- Continued													
044	Illinois Central College Ms Mary Beth Kiefner, Supv *Chair's #: (309) 999-4600*	201 SW Adams East Peoria	61635			A	CC	PBL	11	12	12	12	11	12
051	Illinois Valley Comm College Mrs Bonnie Grusk, Dir *Chair's #: (815) 224-2720 Ext 485*	815 Orlando Smith Ave Oglesby	61348				CC	PBL	11	12	15	20	21	17
035	Jacksnvl Sch of PN-Bd of Ed-Dist 117 Ms Joan Ortman, Dir *Chair's #: (217) 245-9225*	49 N Central Park Plaza Jacksonville	62650				SEC	PVT	11	12	25	33	26	27
048	John A Logan College Mrs Debra Goddard, Dir *Chair's #: (618) 985-3741 Ext 455*	RR #2 Carterville	62918				CC	PBL	12	12	62	70	89	69
022	John Wood Comm College-PN Mrs Sandra McKelvie, Director *Chair's #: (217) 224-6500 Ext 4550*	150 S 48th St Quincy	62301				CC	PBL			53	51	35	27
031	Joliet Township HS Mrs Arthetta Reeder, Dir *Chair's #: (815) 727-6885*	201 E Jefferson Joliet	60432				TCH	PBL	11	12	41	56	44	54
033	Kankakee Comm College Mrs Phyllis Nichols, Director *Chair's #: (815) 933-0295*	Box 888 River Dr Kankakee	60901				CC	PBL			Publication withheld			
055	Kaskaskia College Mrs Marylou Whitten, Dir *Chair's #: (618) 532-1981 Ext 332*	27210 College Rd Centralia	62801				CC	PBL	11	12	25	25	16	30
042	Kishwaukee College-PN Sch Ms Heather Peters, Dir *Chair's #: (815) 825-2086 Ext 355*	21193 Malta Rd Malta	60150		7			CC	PBL			Data reported w/AD Prog			
016	Lake Land College Kathleen Doehring, Dir *Chair's #: (217) 234-5204*	5501 Lake Land Blvd Mattoon	61938			A	CC	PBL	12	12	34	39	27	36
061	Lewis And Clark Comm Coll Dr Linda Harner, Coord *Chair's #: (618) 466-3411 Ext 4431*	5800 Godfrey Rd Godfrey	62035				CC	PBL	12	12	11	19	16	11
006	Lincolnland Comm College Ms Joan Lewis, Dept Chair *Chair's #: (217) 786-2200*	Shephard Rd Springfield	62794				CC	PBL			Class Yet To be Admitted			
059	Morton College Mrs Aline Tupa, Coord *Chair's #: (708) 656-8000*	3801 South Central Ave Cicero	60804		7			CC	PBL			Data reported w/AD Prog			

School Code	Name of School, Director of Program, and Phone Number	Street Address / City or Town and Zip Code		Footnotes	Type of Program	NLNAC Accreditation as of January 31, 1998	Administrative Control	Financial Support (principal source)	Number of Months in Program	Educational Requirements for Entering Adult Program	Enrollments as of October 15, 1997	Admissions Aug. 1, 1996 - July 31, 1997	Graduations Aug. 1, 1996 - July 31, 1997	Fall Admissions Aug. 1, 1997 - Dec. 31, 1997
	ILLINOIS													
	- Continued													
047	Oakton Comm College Ms Marilou Wasseluk, Chair *Chair's #: (847) 635-1720*	1600 East Golf Road Des Plaines	60016				CC	PBL			23	27	23	0
050	Parkland College Practical Nsg Program Dr Sharon A Gerth, Chair *Chair's #: (217) 351-2289*	2400 W Bradley Ave Champaign	61821			A	CC	PBL	12	12	15	22	12	16
023	Rend Lake College Ms Wilanna Patton, Chair *Chair's #: (618) 437-5321 Ext 225*	Ina	62846				CC	PBL			Publication withheld			
019	Rockford School of Practical Nursing Mrs S Carlson Asher, Dir *Chair's #: (815) 906-3716*	978 Haskell Ave Rockford	61103			A	SEC	PBL	11	12	27	45	43	27
026	Sauk Valley Comm Coll Ms Rosemary Johnson, Director *Chair's #: (815) 288-5511 Ext 376*	173 Illinois Route #2 Dixon	61021				CC	PBL			16	19	12	18
043	Shawnee Comm College Dr Jeannine Hayduk, Dir *Chair's #: (618) 634-2242 Ext 200*	Rt 1 Box 53 Ullin	62992				CC	PBL			Publication withheld			
046	South Suburban College Ms Judith A Coglianese, Exec Dir *Chair's #: (708) 596-2000 Ext 2260*	15800 S State St South Holland	60473			A	CC	PBL	11	12	49	47	30	50
012	Southeastern Illinois College Mrs Nancy Buttry, Dir *Chair's #: (618) 252-5400 Ext 2331*	3575 College Rd Harrisburg	62946				CC	PBL			123	120	82	102
045	Spoon River College Ms Janis Waite, Assoc Dean *Chair's #: (309) 647-4645 Ext 333*	23235 N County 22 Canton	61520	7			CC	PBL			Data Reported w/AD Prog			
039	Triton College Mrs Sharon Abbate, Chair *Chair's #: (708) 456-0300 Ext 3656*	2000 5th Ave River Grove	60171			A	CC	PBL	18	12	95	110	91	50
041	William Rainey Harper College Mrs Cheryl Wandambi, Dir *Chair's #: (847) 925-6683*	1200 West Algonquin Rd Palatine	60067	7			CC	PBL			Data reported w/AD prog			
	INDIANA													
	22 Programs in 22 Schools													
016	Anderson PN Sch-Anderson Comm Schs Mrs Marcia Scott, Dir *Chair's #: (765) 683-3015*	325 W 38th St Anderson	46013				TCH	PBL	12	12	36	39	51	20

Explanation of footnotes on page x

School Code	Name of School, Director of Program, and Phone Number	Street Address City or Town and Zip Code	Footnotes	Type of Program	NLNAC Accreditation as of January 31, 1998	Administrative Control	Financial Support (principal source)	Number of Months in Program	Educational Requirements for Entering Adult Program	Enrollments as of October 15, 1997	Admissions Aug. 1, 1996 - July 31, 1997	Graduations Aug. 1, 1996 - July 31, 1997	Fall Admissions Aug. 1, 1997 - Dec. 31, 1997
	INDIANA												
	- Continued												
031	Horizon Career College Ms Cristine O'Brien , Coord *Chair's #: (219) 756-6811*	8315 Virginia St Suite A Merrillville 46410				CC	PBL			Publication withheld			
018	Indiana V-T College Sch of PN, Reg 1 Mrs Karen Warner, Chair *Chair's #: (219) 464-8514 Ext 25*	2401 Valley Dr Valparaiso 46383			A	TCH	PBL			100	90	75	60
013	Indiana V-T College Sch of PN, Reg 10 Ms Celinda K Leach, Chair *Chair's #: (812) 332-1559 Ext 4325*	3116 Canterbury Ct Bloomington 47402				TCH	PBL	12	12	63	66	50	40
020	Indiana V-T College Sch of PN, Reg 2 Mrs Gene Ann Shapinsky, Chair *Chair's #: (812) 265-2580 Ext 4167*	Hwy 62 & Ivy Tech Dr Madison 47250				TCH	PBL	12	12	52	60	50	53
005	Indiana V-T College Sch of PN, Reg 2 Mrs Donna Keusch, Chair *Chair's #: (219) 236-7173 Ext 720*	1534 W Sample St South Bend 46619				TCH	PBL	12	12	124	91	71	73
008	Indiana V-T College Sch of PN, Reg 7 Mrs Leota Ehm, Chair *Chair's #: (812) 299-1121 Ext 287*	7377 SO Dixie Bee Rd Terre Haute 47802				CC	PBL	12	12	101	100	84	51
002	Indiana V-T College Sch of PN, Reg 7 Mrs Lucy White, Chair *Chair's #: (765) 653-7410*	12 North Jackson Greencastle 46135				TCH	PBL	17	12	26	30	19	30
011	Indiana V-T College Sch of PN, Reg 9 Mrs Jillene Anderson, Chair *Chair's #: (765) 983-3210*	1401 Chester Blvd Richmond 47374				TCH	PBL	12	12	81	97	70	96
024	Indiana Voc Tech College Mrs Elaine Schmidt, Chair *Chair's #: (812) 429-1453*	3501 First Ave Evansville 47710			A	TCH	PBL	12	12	47	64	49	47
017	IVTC , Reg 4 Mrs Marsha Duda, Chair *Chair's #: (765)-772-9100*	3208 Ross Rd PO Box 6299 Lafayette 47903				TCH	PBL			Publication withheld			
900	IVY Tech State Coll Ms Peggy Riley, Chair *Chair's #: (317) 289-2291 Ext 341*	4301 South Cowan Rd Muncie 47302				CC	PBL			Publication withheld			
009	IVY Tech State Coll -Hlth Tech State Co Ms Geneva Lamm, Chair *Chair's #: (812) 372-9925 Ext 134*	4475 Central Ave Columbus 47203				TCH	PBL	12	12	99	78	75	0
010	Ivy Tech State Coll Reg 13 Ms Sue Jewell, Chair *Chair's #: (812) 246-3301 Ext 4195*	8204 Hwy 311 Sellersburg 47172				TCH	PBL			58	70	50	58

Explanation of footnotes on page x

School Code	Name of School, Director of Program, and Phone Number	Street Address City or Town and Zip Code	Footnotes	Type of Program	NLNAC Accreditation as of January 31, 1998	Administrative Control	Financial Support (principal source)	Number of Months in Program	Educational Requirements for Entering Adult Program	Enrollments as of October 15, 1997	Admissions Aug. 1, 1996 - July 31, 1997	Graduations Aug. 1, 1996 - July 31, 1997	Fall Admissions Aug. 1, 1997 - Dec. 31, 1997
	INDIANA												
	- Continued												
006	IVY Tech State Coll Reg 3 Mrs JoAnn Dever, Chair *Chair's #: (219) 480-4272*	3800 N Anthony Blvd Fort Wayne 46805				TCH	PBL	12	12	229	140	125	70
030	IVY Tech State Coll-Reg 5 Mrs Gerry Mooney, Chair *Chair's #: (317) 459-0561 Ext 427*	1815 E Morgan Box 1373 Kokomo 46903				GOV	PBL			Publication withheld			
023	IVY Tech State College Ms Saundra Horne, Chair *Chair's #: (219) 981-4412*	1440 East 35th Ave Gary 46409				TCH	PBL	12	12	72	58	40	0
001	Ivy Tech State College Ms Barbara Deady, Chair *Chair's #: (317) 921-4407*	One West 26th St Box 1763 Indianapolis 46206			A	TCH	PBL	12	12	119	140	112	70
019	J E Light Sch of PN Metro Sch Dist Mrs Karen Selwa Williams, Dir *Chair's #: (317) 259-5265 Ext 4017*	1901 E 86 St Indianapolis 46240				TCH	PBL			Publication withheld			
004	Marion Comm Sch-Tuckr Area V-T Ctr Ms Joyce Dolby, Dir *Chair's #: (765) 664-9091*	107 S Pennsylvania Ave Marion 46952				TCH	PBL	12	12	28	32	21	32
029	St Anthony Medical Center Ms Carol Anderson, Director *Chair's #: (219) 757-6406 Ext 6406*	203 Franciscan Dr Crown Point 46307				HSP	PVT			Publication withheld			
015	Vincennes Univ, Practical Nsg Program Ms Karen R Gines, Chair *Chair's #: (812) 888-4325*	1002 North First St Vincennes 47591			A	CC	PBL	11	12	25	32	23	30
021	Vincennes Univ-Jasper Campus Mrs Mary Price, Director *Chair's #: (812) 481-5926*	850 College Ave Jasper 47546			A	CC	PBL	13	12	16	18	15	18
	IOWA												
	29 Programs in 18 Schools												
028	BVU-Iowa Central Comm College Mrs Brenda Gleason, Dir *Chair's #: (515) 576-7201 Ext 2310*	620 W 4th St Bx 2020 Storm Lake 50588	7			CC	PBL			Data reported w/AD prog			
012	Des Moines Area Comm Coll-Boone Ms Susan Wager, Director *Chair's #: (515) 964-6316*	1125 Hancock Dr Boone 50036			A	CC	PBL	9	12	39	38	35	39
006	Des Moines Area Comm College-Anken Ms Susan Wager, Director *Chair's #: (515) 964-6316*	2006 Ankeny Blvd Bldg 9 Ankeny 50021			A	CC	PBL	9	12	72	75	57	75

Explanation of footnotes on page x

School Code	Name of School, Director of Program, and Phone Number	Street Address / City or Town and Zip Code		Footnotes	Type of Program	NLNAC Accreditation as of January 31, 1998	Administrative Control	Financial Support (principal source)	Number of Months in Program	Educational Requirements for Entering Adult Program	Enrollments as of October 15, 1997	Admissions Aug. 1, 1996 - July 31, 1997	Graduations Aug. 1, 1996 - July 31, 1997	Fall Admissions Aug. 1, 1997 - Dec. 31, 1997
	IOWA													
	- Continued													
007	Des Moines Area Comm College-Carroll Ms Susan Wager, Director *Chair's #: (515) 964-6316*	906 N Grant Rd Carroll	51401			A	CC	PBL	9	12	26	28	20	28
026	Des Moines Central Campus Mrs Martha A Schaer, Coord *Chair's #: (515) 242-7846 Ext 3462*	1800 Grand Ave Des Moines	50309				SEC	PBL			25	17	10	12
009	Eastern Iowa CC Dist-Clinton CC Ms Nancy E Knutstrom, Coord *Chair's #: (319) 242-6841 Ext 384*	1000 Lincoln Blvd Clinton	52732				CC	PBL			Publication withheld			
008	Eastern Iowa CC Dist-Scott CC Ms Nancy E Knutstrom, Coord *Chair's #: (319) 359-7531 Ext 304*	500 Belmont Rd Bettendorf	52722				CC	PBL			Publication withheld			
005	Hawkeye Comm College Mrs Brenda Berry, Coord *Chair's #: (319) 296-2320 Ext 4013*	1501 E Orange Rd Box 8015 Waterloo	50704				CC	PBL			Publication withheld			
010	Indian Hills CC-Ottumwa Ms M Ann Aulwes, Chair *Chair's #: (515) 683-5165 Ext 5165*	525 Grandview Ottumwa	52501				CC	PBL	13	12	57	77	49	0
014	Indian Hills Comm College-Centerville Ms M Ann Aulwes, Chair *Chair's #: (515) 683-5111 Ext 5165*	721 N First St Centerville	52544				CC	PBL			Publication withheld			
031	Iowa Central CC-Webster City Mrs Diane Sorensen, Coord *Chair's #: (515) 832-1632*	1725 Beach St Webster City	50595		7			CC	PBL			Data reported w/AD prog			
021	Iowa Central Comm College-Fort Dodge Mrs Brenda Gleason, Dir *Chair's #: (515) 576-0099 Ext 2310*	330 Ave M Fort Dodge	50501				CC	PBL	10	12	11	10	29	12
015	Iowa Lakes Comm College Mrs Judi Donahue, Dir *Chair's #: (712) 852-5285*	3200 College Ave Emmetsburg	50536		7			CC	PBL			Data reported w/AD prog			
001	Iowa Valley Comm College (2 Campus Mrs Mavis A Hunt, Coord *Chair's #: (515) 752-7106 Ext 297*	3700 S Center St Marshalltown	50158				CC	PBL			Publication withheld			
004	Iowa Western Comm College-Clarinda Roberta Kokenge, Coord *Chair's #: (712) 542-5117 Ext 240*	923 E Washington Clarinda	51632				CC	PBL	11	12	32	36	32	0
019	Iowa Western Comm College-Council Bl Mrs Karen Sojka, Assoc Dean *Chair's #: (712) 325-3200 Ext 352*	2700 College Rd Box 4-C Council Bluffs	51502		7			TCH	PBL			Data reported w/AD prog			

Explanation of footnotes on page x

School Code	Name of School, Director of Program, and Phone Number	Street Address / City or Town and Zip Code	Footnotes	Type of Program	NLNAC Accreditation as of January 31, 1998	Administrative Control	Financial Support (principal source)	Number of Months in Program	Educational Requirements for Entering Adult Program	Enrollments as of October 15, 1997	Admissions Aug. 1, 1996 - July 31, 1997	Graduations Aug. 1, 1996 - July 31, 1997	Fall Admissions Aug. 1, 1997 - Dec. 31, 1997
	IOWA												
	- Continued												
027	Iowa Western Comm College-Harlan Ms Sue Smith, Coord *Chair's #: (712) 755-3568*	2712 12th St Harlan 51537				CC	PBL	12	12	12	33	16	0
017	Kirkwood Comm College Ms Linda Schwartz, Coord *Chair's #: (319) 398-5630*	6301 Kirkwood Blvd SW Bx 20 Cedar Rapids 52406	7			CC	PBL			Data reported w/AD prog			
011	North Iowa Area Comm College Mrs Donna J Orton, Chair *Chair's #: (515) 421-4216*	500 College Dr Mason City 50401	7			CC	PBL	11	12	15	22	11	0
023	Northeast Iowa Comm Coll-Calmar Mrs Melinda Hanson, Chair *Chair's #: (319) 562-3263 Ext 262*	Box 400 Hwy 150 South Calmar 52132	7			CC	PBL			Datareported w/ADprog			
020	Northeast Iowa Comm Coll-Peosta Mrs Geraldine Althoff, Dir *Chair's #: (319) 556-5110 Ext 209*	10250 Sundown Rd Peosta 52068				CC	PBL			Publication withheld			
030	Northwest Iowa Comm College Mrs Mary C Mohni, Dir *Chair's #: (712) 324-5061 Ext 117*	Hwy 18 West Sheldon 51201				CC	PBL	11	12	34	37	25	37
016	Southeastern Comm College-Burlington Mrs Anita M Stineman, Admin *Chair's #: (319) 752-2731 Ext 8164*	1015 S Gear Ave West Burlington 52655				CC	PBL	12	12	9	13	28	0
029	Southeastern Comm College-Keokuk Mrs Anita M Stineman, Admin *Chair's #: (319) 524-3221 Ext 8442*	335 Messenger Rd Box 6007 Keokuk 52632				CC	PBL	12	12	6	14	15	0
024	Southwestern Comm College Mrs Loretta A Eckels, Chair *Chair's #: (515) 782-7081 Ext 271*	1501 Townline St Creston 50801				CC	PBL			Publication withheld			
013	Western Iowa Tech Comm Coll (3 Camp Dr Gloria Stewart, Div Chair *Chair's #: (712) 274-8733 Ext 1350*	4647 Stone Ave Box 265 Sioux City 51106			A	CC	PBL	9	12	117	148	67	83
	KANSAS												
	18 Programs in 17 Schools												
020	Barton Co Comm College Ms Karla Homan, Director *Chair's #: (316) 792-9355*	Great Bend 67530				CC	PBL	11	12	32	37	21	37
021	Butler Co Comm College Ms Patricia Bayles, Dean *Chair's #: (316) 322-3146*	901 S Haverhill Rd El Dorado 67042	7			CC	PBL			Data reported w/AD prog			

Explanation of footnotes on page x

School Code	Name of School, Director of Program, and Phone Number	Street Address / City or Town and Zip Code		Footnotes	Type of Program	NLNAC Accreditation as of January 31, 1998	Administrative Control	Financial Support (principal source)	Number of Months in Program	Educational Requirements for Entering Adult Program	Enrollments as of October 15, 1997	Admissions Aug. 1, 1996 - July 31, 1997	Graduations Aug. 1, 1996 - July 31, 1997	Fall Admissions Aug. 1, 1997 - Dec. 31, 1997
	KANSAS													
	- Continued													
012	Colby Community College Mrs Janet Myers, Dir *Chair's #: (785) 462-4788 Ext 319*	1255 S Range Colby	67701	7			A	CC	PBL			Data reported w/AD prog			
005	Dodge City Community College Mrs Linda K Sanko, Director *Chair's #: (316) 225-1321 Ext 226*	2501 N 14th Ave Dodge City	67801				A	CC	PBL	10	12	37	39	34	38
008	Flint Hills Tech Coll Mrs Kathleen Bode, Chair *Chair's #: (316) 341-2300 Ext 226*	3301 W 18th Emporia	66801					TCH	PBL	11	12	40	48	45	24
027	Hutchinson Comm Coll Ms Brenda Lawrence, Dir *Chair's #: (316) 241-4417*	925 N Walnut McPherson	67460				A	CC	PBL	10	12	29	54	29	30
007	Johnson County Comm College/AVS Dr Ann Hess, Coord *Chair's #: (913) 469-2349*	10000 W 75 N St Suite 241 Merriam	66204					CC	PBL			23	24	21	24
016	Kansas City, KS Area Voc-Tech Sch Ms Susan White, Supv *Chair's #: (913) 596-5500 Ext 332*	2220 N 59th St Kansas City	66104					TCH	PBL	11	12	69	101	69	52
004	KAW Area Tech School-Dept of PN Dr Julie Putnam, Coord *Chair's #: (785) 273-7140 Ext 6308*	5724 Huntoon Topeka	66604		HSE		A A	TCH TCH	PBL PBL	10 10	12 12	69 0	61 0	69 0	45 0
022	Labette Comm College Dr W Maxson-Ladage, Assoc Dean *Chair's #: (316) 421-6700 Ext 62*	200 South 14th St Parsons	67357	7				CC	PBL	12	12	43	45	34	45
011	Manhattan Area Tech Coll Mrs Myrna J Bartel, Coord *Chair's #: (785) 587-2800 Ext 121*	3136 Dickens Manhattan	66503					TCH	PBL	11	12	42	45	33	44
006	Neosho County Comm Jr College Ms Carol Fox, Dir *Chair's #: (316) 431-2820 Ext 255*	800 Comm West 14th st Chanute	66720	7				CC	PBL			Data reported with/AD pro			
013	No Ctrl KS Cloud Co Comm Coll Mrs Vera Streit, Coord *Chair's #: (913) 738-2419*	Box 507 Beloit	67420				A	TCH	PBL			Publication withheld			
014	Northeast Kansas Area Tech Sch Ms Janean Bowen, Supv *Chair's #: (913) 367-6204*	1501 W Riley Atchison	66002					TCH	PBL	11	12	30	30	27	0
023	Pratt Comm College Mrs Donna Bauer, Dean *Chair's #: (316) 672-5641 Ext 232*	348 NE State Rd 61 Pratt	67124	7				CC	PBL			Data reported w/AD prog			

School Code	Name of School, Director of Program, and Phone Number	Street Address / City or Town and Zip Code		Footnotes	Type of Program	NLNAC Accreditation as of January 31, 1998	Administrative Control	Financial Support (principal source)	Number of Months in Program	Educational Requirements for Entering Adult Program	Enrollments as of October 15, 1997	Admissions Aug. 1, 1996 - July 31, 1997	Graduations Aug. 1, 1996 - July 31, 1997	Fall Admissions Aug. 1, 1997 - Dec. 31, 1997
	KANSAS													
	- Continued													
019	Seward County Community College Mr Steve Hecox, Chair *Chair's #: (316) 626-3026*	Box 1137 Liberal	67901			A	CC	PBL	10	12	25	25	23	25
003	Wichita Area Tech College Mrs Donna Granger, Specialist *Chair's #: (316) 833-4370*	324 N Emporia Wichita	67202			A	TCH	PBL	12	12	62	66	47	34
	KENTUCKY													
	24 Programs in 18 Schools													
021	Ashland Area Voc School Ms Vicki Hemlepp, Coord *Chair's #: (606) 928-6427 Ext 261*	4818 Roberts Dr Ashland	41101			TCH		PBL	15	12	19	33	21	0
016	Cumberland Vly Hlth Occup Center Mrs Margaret Peace, Admin *Chair's #: (606) 337-3106 Ext 0020*	US 25E Box 187 Pineville	40977			TCH		PBL	15	12	83	69	45	42
007	Danville Hlth Tech Center Mrs Sandra Houston, Director *Chair's #: (606) 239-7030*	1714 Perryville Rd Danville	40423			TCH		PBL	15	12	105	139	73	26
900	Galen Health Inst Mrs Margaret Stutzenberger, Dir *Chair's #: (502) 580-3660*	612 S Fourth Ave Louisville	40202			TCH		PVT	12	12	89	141	83	64
009	Glasgow School for Hlth Occup Mrs Rebecca S Forrest, Director *Chair's #: (502) 651-5673*	129 State Ave Glasgow	42141			TCH		PBL			Publication withheld			
019	Hazard Reg Tech Center Mrs Phyllis Morris, Dept Chair *Chair's #: (606) 435-6101 Ext 166*	101 Vo-Tech Drive Hazard	41701			TCH		PBL	15	12	75	80	37	38
010	Jefferson State Voc-Tech Sch Mrs Jane A Hudson, Coord *Chair's #: (502) 595-4275*	800 W Chestnut St Louisville	40203		HSE	TCH TCH		PBL PBL	15 9	12 12	70 7	80 9	41 8	20 8
004	KY Tech Central Campus Ms Bonnie Nicholson, Chair *Chair's #: (606) 246-2400*	308 Voc Tech Rd Lexington	40511			TCH		PBL			Publication withheld			
015	KY Tech-Owensboro Campus Mrs Nancy Turner, Chair *Chair's #: (502) 687-7273 Ext 147*	1501 Frederica St Owensboro	42301			TCH		PBL	15	12	20	20	17	0
051	KY Tech-Somerset Reg Tech Center Mrs Doris Ball Childers, Coord *Chair's #: (606) 677-4049 Ext 121*	230 Airport Rd Somerset	42501			TCH		PBL		12	30	39	21	30

Explanation of footnotes on page x

School Code	Name of School, Director of Program, and Phone Number	Street Address / City or Town and Zip Code		Footnotes	Type of Program	NLNAC Accreditation as of January 31, 1998	Administrative Control	Financial Support (principal source)	Number of Months in Program	Educational Requirements for Entering Adult Program	Enrollments as of October 15, 1997	Admissions Aug. 1, 1996 - July 31, 1997	Graduations Aug. 1, 1996 - July 31, 1997	Fall Admissions Aug. 1, 1997 - Dec. 31, 1997
	KENTUCKY													
	- Continued													
001	KY Technical-Elizabethtown Mrs Maurita Roper, Coord Chair's #: (502) 766-5133 Ext 163	505 University Dr Elizabethtown	42701				TCH	PBL	15	12	21	0	15	22
020	Madisonville Hlth Tech Center Mrs Clara S Dorris, Coord Chair's #: (502) 824-7552 Ext 165	750 N Laffoon St Madisonville	42431				TCH	PBL	12	12	27	56	59	32
006	Mayo Reg Tech Center (2 Campuses) Ms Sue Garland, Dept Chair Chair's #: (606) 789-5324 Ext 246	W 3rd St Paintsville	41240				TCH	PBL	15		40	33	33	33
022	Murray School of PN Ms Joyce Morrison, Coord Chair's #: (502) 753-1870	18th & Sycamore Murray	42071				TCH	PBL			Publication withheld			
018	No KY Hlth Technology Center Ms Georgianne Duffy, Coord Chair's #: (606) 341-5200	790 Thomas More Parkway Edgewood	41017				TCH	PBL	15	12	30	31	50	27
053	Rowan State Voc Tech Sch of PN (2 Ca Mrs Claudia Collins, Coord Chair's #: (606) 783-1538 Ext 305	100 Vo-Tech Dr Morehead	40351				TCH	PBL	15	12	39	64	32	0
049	Spencerian College Mrs Natalie Hall, Dir Chair's #: (502) 447-1000 Ext 213	4627 Dixie Highway Louisville	40216				IND	PVT	12	12	157	157	107	37
023	West KY St Voc Tech Sch of PN Mrs Marie Thieleman, Coord Chair's #: (502) 554-6270	Box 7408 5200 Blandville Rd Paducah	42002				TCH	PBL	15	12	12	23	18	0
	LOUISIANA													
	48 Programs in 46 Schools													
065	Cameron College Dr Lynn Tarzetti, Dir Chair's #: (504) 821-5881	2740 Canal St New Orleans	70119				CC	PVT			Publication withheld			
052	Delgado Comm Coll Mrs Pearlette Carter, Dir Chair's #: (504) 483-4666 Ext 4646	980 Navarre Ave New Orleans	70124				TCH	PBL	16	12	38	57	33	0
082	Delta College of Arts and Technology Mrs Barbara Demarest, Coord Chair's #: (504) 927-7780 Ext 14	7290 Exchange Pl Baton Rouge	70806				TCH	PVT	15	12	58	31	22	36
047	Elaine P Nunez Comm College Ms Andrea Phillipi, Coord Chair's #: (504) 278-7440	3700 La Fontaine St Chalmette	70043				TCH	PBL			37	40	32	0

School Code	Name of School, Director of Program, and Phone Number	Street Address, City or Town and Zip Code	Footnotes	Type of Program	NLNAC Accreditation as of January 31, 1998	Administrative Control	Financial Support (principal source)	Number of Months in Program	Educational Requirements for Entering Adult Program	Enrollments as of October 15, 1997	Admissions Aug. 1, 1996 - July 31, 1997	Graduations Aug. 1, 1996 - July 31, 1997	Fall Admissions Aug. 1, 1997 - Dec. 31, 1997
	LOUISIANA - Continued												
068	LA Tech Coll Mansfield Campus Ms Camillia Spilker, Coord Chair's #: (318) 872-2243	PO Box 1236 Mansfield 71052				TCH	PBL			26	26	22	0
007	LA Tech Coll-Delta-Ouachita Campus Mrs Paula Ott Nisbet, Dept Head Chair's #: (318) 726-6258 Ext 221	609 Vocational Pky West Monroe 71291				TCH	PBL			Publication withheld			
055	LA Tech Coll-Evangeline Campus Mrs Etta Ramona Hamilton, Coord Chair's #: (318) 394-6466 Ext 19	PO Box 68 St Martinville 70582				TCH	PBL			Publication withheld			
046	LA Tech Coll-Florida Pariches Mr George Foster, Dir Chair's #: (504) 222-4351	PO Box 130 Greensburg 70441				TCH	PBL			Publication withheld			
043	LA Tech Coll-Folkes Campus Mrs Faith Rohner, Dir Chair's #: (504) 342-6661	PO Box 808 Jackson 70748				TCH	PBL	15	12	12	24	15	0
022	LA Tech Coll-Gulf Area Campus Mrs Amy M Sellers, Dept Head Chair's #: (318) 893-4984	PO Box 878 Abbeville 70510				TCH	PBL	16	12	18	35	27	0
020	LA Tech Coll-Hammond Area Campus Mrs Roberta Connelley, Coord Chair's #: (504) 543-4120	PO Box 489 Hammond 70404				TCH	PBL	16	12	28	46	0	0
036	LA Tech Coll-Huey P Long Campus Mrs Evelyn Hyde, Dept Head Chair's #: (318) 628-4342	303 S Jones St Winnfield 71483				TCH	PBL	16	12	43	62	45	0
018	LA Tech Coll-Jefferson Campus Mrs Sandra Dawes, Coord Chair's #: (504) 736-7086	5200 Blair Dr Metairie 70001				TCH	PBL	16	12	76	91	70	0
056	LA Tech Coll-Jefferson Davis Campus Mr Johnnie Smith, Dir Chair's #: (318) 824-4811	PO Box 1327 1230 N Main St Jenning 70546				TCH	PBL	16	12	35	35	17	35
050	LA Tech Coll-Lafayette Campus Mrs Pemella Williams, Dept Head Chair's #: (318) 262-5962	PO Box 4909 Lafayette 70502				TCH	PBL			Publication withheld			
062	LA Tech Coll-Lafourche Campus Mrs Myra Cheramie, Dept Head Chair's #: (504) 447-0924	1425 Tiger Dr Box 1831 Thibodaux 70302				TCH	PBL			Publication withheld			
045	LA Tech Coll-Lamar Salter Campus Ms Patricia Nunnally, Coord Chair's #: (318) 537-3135	15014 Lake Charles Hwy Leesville 71446				TCH	PBL	16	12	22	38	19	0

Explanation of footnotes on page x

School Code	Name of School, Director of Program, and Phone Number	Street Address	City or Town and Zip Code	Footnotes	Type of Program	NLNAC Accreditation as of January 31, 1998	Administrative Control	Financial Support (principal source)	Number of Months in Program	Educational Requirements for Entering Adult Program	Enrollments as of October 15, 1997	Admissions Aug. 1, 1996 - July 31, 1997	Graduations Aug. 1, 1996 - July 31, 1997	Fall Admissions Aug. 1, 1997 - Dec. 31, 1997
	LOUISIANA													
	- Continued													
024	LA Tech Coll-Natchitoches Campus Mrs Melanie McMillin, Coord *Chair's #: (318) 357-3162*	PO Box 657	Natchitoches 71457				TCH	PBL			25	37	19	0
035	LA Tech Coll-Northeast LA Campus Mrs Beverly Peoples, Coord *Chair's #: (318) 435-2163*	1710 Warren St	Winnsboro 71295				TCH	PBL	18	11	15	33	21	3
044	LA Tech Coll-Northwest LA Campus Mrs Sharon Turley, Dept Head *Chair's #: (318) 927-3035*	PO Box 835	Minden 71058				TCH	PBL			Publication withheld			
058	LA Tech Coll-Oakdale Campus Mrs Rebecca Harrell, Coord *Chair's #: (318) 335-3944*	PO Drawer E M	Oakdale 71463				TCH	PBL			Publication withheld			
042	LA Tech Coll-Ruston Campus Mrs Janet Armstrong, Instructor *Chair's #: (318) 251-4145*	PO Box 1070	Ruston 71273				TCH	PBL	14	12	73	46	28	0
001	LA Tech Coll-Shreveport-Bossier Camp Mrs Ann Caskey Ryals, Coord *Chair's #: (318) 676-7811*	2010 N Market St	Shreveport 71107				TCH	PBL			Publication withheld			
028	La Tech Coll-Sidney N Collins Campus Mrs Desaree Holmes, Dept Head *Chair's #: (504) 942-8333*	3727 Louisa St	New Orleans 70126				TCH	PBL			70	103	62	0
034	LA Tech Coll-Slidell Campus Mrs Barbara Holloway, Dept Head *Chair's #: (504) 646-6430 Ext 52*	PO Box 827	Slidell 70459				TCH	PBL	18	12	15	29	0	45
025	LA Tech Coll-South LA Campus Mrs Donna Leach Kane, Dept Head *Chair's #: (504) 857-3655*	PO Box 5033	Houma 70361				TCH	PBL	15	12	40	60	42	0
006	La Tech Coll-Sowela Campus Mrs Phyllis Robinson, Dept Head *Chair's #: (318) 491-2696*	3820 Legion St	Lake Charles 70601				TCH	PBL			Publication withheld			
015	LA Tech Coll-Sullivan Campus Ms Judy Wamsley, Dept Head *Chair's #: (504) 732-6640 Ext 23*	1710 Sullivan Dr	Bogalusa 70427				TCH	PBL			Publication withheld			
012	LA Tech Coll-T H Harris Campus Mrs Laurie Fontenot, Dept Head *Chair's #: (318) 948-0336*	PO Box 713	Opelousas 70570				TCH	PBL	15	12	75	108	32	50
049	LA Tech Coll-Tallulah Campus Mrs Margaret Shoemaker, Coord *Chair's #: (318) 574-4820 Ext 0007*	PO Drawer 1740	Tallulah 71282				TCH	PBL			Publication withheld			

School Code	Name of School, Director of Program, and Phone Number	Street Address, City or Town and Zip Code		Footnotes	Type of Program	NLNAC Accreditation as of January 31, 1998	Administrative Control	Financial Support (principal source)	Number of Months in Program	Educational Requirements for Entering Adult Program	Enrollments as of October 15, 1997	Admissions Aug. 1, 1996 - July 31, 1997	Graduations Aug. 1, 1996 - July 31, 1997	Fall Admissions Aug. 1, 1997 - Dec. 31, 1997
	LOUISIANA													
	- Continued													
038	LA Tech Coll-W Jefferson Campus Ms Ruth Finney, Head Chair's #: (504) 361-6471	475 Manhattan Blvd Harvey	70058				TCH	PBL			Publication withheld			
026	LA Tech Coll-Westside Campus Mr Alfred Bell, Dir Chair's #: (504) 687-6392	PO Box 733 Plaquemine	70764				TCH	PBL	14	12	27	48	0	48
021	LA Tech Coll-Young Memorial Campus Mr Gregory Garrett, Dir Chair's #: (504) 380-2436	PO Box 2148 Morgan City	70380				TCH	PBL			Publication withheld			
066	LA Tech College At Ville Platte Mr Mark A Doucet, Coord Chair's #: (318) 363-2197 Ext 135	PO Box 296 Ville Platte	70586				TCH	PBL	18	12	31	25	22	45
014	LA Tech College-Alexandria Campus Ms Stephanie Jackson, Dept Head Chair's #: (318) 487-5435	4311 S MacArthur Dr Alexandria	71301				TCH	PBL			Publication withheld			
051	LA Tech College-Avoyelles Campus Mrs Kate Moreau, Coord Chair's #: (318) 563-8685	PO Box 307 Cottonport	73127				TCH	PBL	16	12	60	84	45	45
008	LA Tech College-Baton Rouge Campus Ms Beverly W McNeese, Dept Head Chair's #: (504) 342-0573	3250 N Acadian Hwy Baton Rouge	70805				TCH	PBL			0	0	0	0
900	LA Tech College-Clairborne Campus Ms Melinda Parnell, Coord Chair's #: (318) 927-2034	3001 Minden Rd Homer	71050				TCH	PBL			25	36	18	30
004	LA Technical Coll-S Jackson Campus Mrs Mignonne Ater, Coord Chair's #: (318) 757-6501	Po Box 152 Ferriday	71334				TCH	PBL			Publication withheld			
019	LA Technical Coll-Teche Area Campus Ms Vickie Migues, Coord Chair's #: (318) 373-0011	PO Box 1057 New Iberia	70562				TCH	PBL	16		29	86	31	46
016	LA Technical College Mrs Jean Houin, Coord Chair's #: (504) 536-4418 Ext 216	181 Regala Pk Reserve	70084				TCH	PBL	15	12	12	30	15	3
040	LA Technical College Bastrop Ms Tammy Le Bleu, Coord Chair's #: (318) 283-0836 Ext 21	PO Box 1120 Bastrop	71220				TCH	PBL			Publication withheld			
063	LA Technical College-North Central Mr Kenneth Bridges, Dir Chair's #: (318) 368-3179	PO Box 548 Farmerville	71241				TCH	PBL	16	12	15	32	9	0

Explanation of footnotes on page x

School Code	Name of School, Director of Program, and Phone Number	Street Address / City or Town and Zip Code		Footnotes	Type of Program	NLNAC Accreditation as of January 31, 1998	Administrative Control	Financial Support (principal source)	Number of Months in Program	Educational Requirements for Entering Adult Program	Enrollments as of October 15, 1997	Admissions Aug. 1, 1996 - July 31, 1997	Graduations Aug. 1, 1996 - July 31, 1997	Fall Admissions Aug. 1, 1997 - Dec. 31, 1997
	LOUISIANA													
	- Continued													
005	LA-Tech College-Acadian Campus	1933 W Hutchinson Ave					TCH	PVT	15	11	19	35	0	0
	Mrs Rosalyn Z, Baty, Dept Head	Crowley	70526		HS		TCH	PVT		11	16	13	13	16
	Chair's #: (318) 788-7521													
009	Lafayette Gen Med Center	1214 Coolidge					HSP	PVT			24	33	20	0
	Mrs Heidi H Benoit, Coord	Lafayette	70505											
	Chair's #: (318) 289-8446													
048	LTC, Jumonville-Memorial Campus	PO Box 725					TCH	PBL			Publication withheld			
	Mr Tommy Gauthier, Dir	New Roads	70760											
	Chair's #: (504) 638-8613 Ext 12													
	MAINE													
	5 Programs in 5 Schools													
005	Central Maine Tech College	1250 Turner St		7			CC	PBL			Data reported w/AD Prog			
	Ms Anne Schuettinger, Chair	Auburn	04210											
	Chair's #: (207) 784-2385 Ext 408													
006	Eastern Maine Tech College	Hogan Rd		7			TCH	PBL			Data reported w/AD prog			
	Ms Marilyn A Lavelle, Chair	Bangor	04401											
	Chair's #: (207) 941-4600 Ext 4657													
002	Kennebec Valley Tech College	92 Western Ave		7			TCH	PBL			Data reported w/AD Prog			
	Mrs Marcia Parker, Chair	Fairfield	04937											
	Chair's #: (207) 453-5167													
001	Northern Maine Tech College	33 Edgemont Dr		7			TCH	PBL			Data reported w/AD Prog			
	Mrs B Kent Conant, Chair	Presque Isle	04769											
	Chair's #: (207) 768-2749													
003	Southern Maine Tech College	Fort Rd		7			CC	PBL			Data reported w/AD prog			
	Mrs Nancy Smith, Chair	South Portland	04106											
	Chair's #: (207) 767-9590													
	MARYLAND													
	11 Programs in 11 Schools													
043	Allegany Coll of Maryland	12401 Willowbrook Rd		7			CC	PBL			Data reported w/AD prog			
	Mrs Fran Leibfreid, Dir	Cumberland	21502											
	Chair's #: (301) 784-5568													
017	Baltimore City Public Sch-PN	4501 Edmoson Ave					SEC	PBL	24		0	0	0	0
	Ms Barbara Kinder, Nurse Admin	Baltimore	21229		HS		SEC	PBL		10	28	24	0	15
	Chair's #: (410) 396-7267													
036	Carroll County Career & Tech Center						SEC	PBL	12	12	7	7	13	7
	Mrs Catherine Engel, Principal	Westminster	21157		HS		SEC	PBL	12	12	7	15	5	7
	Chair's #: (410) 751-3669													
050	Cecil Comm College	1000 North East Rd		7			CC	PBL			Data reported w/AD prog			
	Mrs Mary Way Bolt, Dir	North East	21901											
	Chair's #: (410) 287-6060 Ext 333													

Explanation of footnotes on page x

School Code	Name of School, Director of Program, and Phone Number	Street Address, City or Town and Zip Code	Footnotes	Type of Program	NLNAC Accreditation as of January 31, 1998	Administrative Control	Financial Support (principal source)	Number of Months in Program	Educational Requirements for Entering Adult Program	Enrollments as of October 15, 1997	Admissions Aug. 1, 1996 - July 31, 1997	Graduations Aug. 1, 1996 - July 31, 1997	Fall Admissions Aug. 1, 1997 - Dec. 31, 1997
	MARYLAND												
	- Continued												
042	Charles County Community College Ms Margaret DeStafanis, Chair Chair's #: (301) 934-7534	Mitchell Rd, Box 910 La Plata 20646			A	CC	PBL	11	12	18	20	21	19
048	Fredreick Comm Coll PN prog Ms Jane Garvin, Dir Chair's #: (301) 846-2525	7932 Opossumtown Pike Fredrick 21702	7			CC	PBL			Data reported w/AD prog			
044	Harford Comm College PN Prog Mrs Tina Zimmerman, Chair Chair's #: (410) 836-4229	401 Thomas Run Rd Bel Air 21014	7			CC	PBL			Data reported w/AD prog			
051	Howard Comm Coll Dr Emily Slunt, Chair Chair's #: (410) 772-4888	Little Patuyent Pkwy Columbia 21044				CC	PBL	11	12	26	25	28	26
040	PN Program Center for Applied Tech Mrs Mary I Campbell, Admin Chair's #: (410) 544-3616 Ext 206	Stevenson Rd-Rt 7-Bx 265 Severn 21144	HS HSE			SEC SEC SEC	PBL PBL PBL	18 18	10 10	6 48	3 27	5 18	3 27
052	Prince George's Comm Coll Dr Lois Neuman, Chair Chair's #: (301) 322-0734	301 Largo Rd Largo 20774				CC	PBL	12	12	20	20	10	20
045	Wor-Wic Comm College Nsg Dept Ms Denise Marshall, Dept Head Chair's #: (410) 221-2555	Eshc-PO Box 800 Cambridge 21613				CC	PBL			Publication withheld			
	MASSACHUSETTS												
	26 Programs in 21 Schools												
050	Assabet Valley Reg Voc Sch Mrs Joan Kilroy, Coord Chair's #: (508) 485-9430 Ext 471	Fitchburg St Marlboro 01752				TCH	PBL	10	12	39	39	27	40
055	Berkshire Comm College Dr Margaret Chalmers, Chair Chair's #: (413) 499-4660 Ext 450	343 Main St Great Barrington 01230				CC	PBL			Publication withheld			
027	Blue Hills Regional Tech Sch Mrs Maureen McCann, Chair Chair's #: (617) 828-5800 Ext 305	800 Randolph St Canton 02021				TCH	PVT			39	30	28	39
049	Bristol-Plymouth Reg Voc-Tech Sch Mrs Carolyn Pearson, Dir Chair's #: (508) 823-5151 Ext 240	940 County St Taunton 02780				TCH	PBL	10		39	41	34	40
026	Diman Reg Voc-Tech Sch Ms Barbara Pitera, Director Chair's #: (508) 678-2891 Ext 156	Stonehaven Rd Fall River 02723				TCH	PVT	10	12	63	52	46	49

Explanation of footnotes on page x

School Code	Name of School, Director of Program, and Phone Number	Street Address City or Town and Zip Code		Footnotes	Type of Program	NLNAC Accreditation as of January 31, 1998	Administrative Control	Financial Support (principal source)	Number of Months in Program	Educational Requirements for Entering Adult Program	Enrollments as of October 15, 1997	Admissions Aug. 1, 1996 - July 31, 1997	Graduations Aug. 1, 1996 - July 31, 1997	Fall Admissions Aug. 1, 1997 - Dec. 31, 1997
	MASSACHUSETTS													
	- Continued													
029	EATI PN Prog Mrs Donna Lampman, Dept Head *Chair's #: (978) 774-0050 Ext 270*	562 Maple St Hathorne	01937				TCH	PBL	10	12	37	40	29	37
053	Greater Lowell Reg Voc-Tech Sch Ms Nancy Harrington, Dir *Chair's #: (978) 441-0990 Ext 225*	Pawtucket Blvd Tyngsboro	01879				TCH	PVT	10	12	79	80	65	80
028	Greenfield Comm College-PN Prog Ms Virginia Wahl, Coord *Chair's #: (413) 586-9771*	80 Locust St Northampton	01060				CC	PBL	10	12	29	30	28	29
019	Lemuel Shattuck Hosp Sch of PN Dr Mary Keaveny, Dir *Chair's #: (617) 522-8110 Ext 458*	180 Morton St Jamaica Plain	02130				HSP	PBL			Publication withheld			
056	MA Bay Comm College Ms Elleen Andrews O'Brien, Coord *Chair's #: (508) 270-4257*	19 Flagg Drive Framingham	01701				CC	PBL	10	12	82	82	54	85
002	Montachussett RVTS Ms Marjorie Tremblay, Director *Chair's #: (978) 345-9200 Ext 107*	1050 Wesmister St Fitchburgh	01420	1			TCH	PBL			First Class in fall of 98			
054	Northern Essex Comm College Mrs Flora S McLaughlin, Chair *Chair's #: (978) 738-7446*	Elliot Way Haverhill	01830			A	CC	PBL	10	12	37	48	32	39
041	Quincy College Mrs Marybeth Pepin, Chair *Chair's #: (617) 984-1692*	34 Coddington St Quincy	02169			A	CC	PBL			Publication withheld			
001	Shawsheen Valley T H S Mrs Barbara Ahern, Coord *Chair's #: (508) 663-2722 Ext 219*	100 Cook St Billerica	01821				TCH	PBL	10	12	41	42	42	42
020	Soldiers' Home Ms Lorraine T Brown, Director *Chair's #: (617) 884-5660 Ext 627*	91 Crest Ave Chelsea	02150			A	GOV	PBL	11		39	40	31	40
034	Southeastern Reg Voc-Tech Sch Mrs Hilary Hamilton, Director *Chair's #: (508) 230-9241*	250 Foundry St South Easton	02375				TCH	PBL			Publication withheld			
044	Upper Cape Cod Reg Tech Sch Dr Joan Bruce, Coordinator *Chair's #: (508) 759-7711 Ext 285*	220 Sandwich Rd Bourne	02532				TCH	PBL	10		29	30	24	30
037	William J Dean Tech HS Miss Eleanor A Hepburn, Director *Chair's #: (413) 534-2086*	1045 Main St Holyoke	01040				TCH	PBL	10	12	30	30	28	30

School Code	Name of School, Director of Program, and Phone Number	Street Address / City or Town and Zip Code		Footnotes	Type of Program	NLNAC Accreditation as of January 31, 1998	Administrative Control	Financial Support (principal source)	Number of Months in Program	Educational Requirements for Entering Adult Program	Enrollments as of October 15, 1997	Admissions Aug. 1, 1996 - July 31, 1997	Graduations Aug. 1, 1996 - July 31, 1997	Fall Admissions Aug. 1, 1997 - Dec. 31, 1997
	MASSACHUSETTS													
	- Continued													
018	Worcester Tech Inst Mrs Junea M Hutchins, Dept Head *Chair's #: (508) 799-1947*	251 Belmont St Worcester	01605				TCH	PBL			Publication withheld			
007	Youville Hosp Sch of Practical Nursing Ms Helen M Barrett, Director *Chair's #: (617) 964-4144*	15 Walnut Park Newton	02158			A	HSP	PVT	10	12	51	62	50	52
	MICHIGAN													
	27 Programs in 27 Schools													
042	Alpena Comm College Mrs Kathleen McGillis, Asst Dean *Chair's #: (517) 356-9021 Ext 226*	666 Johnson St Alpena	49707	7			CC	PBL			Data reported w/AD prog			
033	Bay de Noc Comm College Mrs Patricia Valensky, Dean *Chair's #: (800) 221-2001 Ext 1208*	2001 North Lincoln Rd Escanaba	49829				CC	PBL	12	12	97	70	62	48
014	Bay Mills Comm Coll Mrs Carol Franklin, Director *Chair's #: (906) 248-5843*	Rt 1 Box 315 A Brinley	49715	1			CC	PBL			Publication withheld			
007	Charles Stewart Mott Comm College Ms Patricia Markowicz, Assoc Dean *Chair's #: (810) 232-3271*	1401 E Court St Flint	48503	7	HSE		CC CC	PBL PBL			Data reported w/AD Prog			
012	Delta College Ms Beth Zieman, Coord *Chair's #: (517) 686-9500*	University Center	48710				CC	PBL			Publication withheld			
036	Glen Oaks Comm College-Div Nsg Ed Mrs Gail Brown, Dir *Chair's #: (616) 467-9945 Ext 247*	62249 Shimmel Rd Centreville	49032				CC	PBL			Publication withheld			
041	Gogebic Comm College Ms Kathryn Encalada, Director *Chair's #: (906) 932-4231 Ext 342*	E 4946 Jackson Rd Ironwood	49938				CC	PBL	11	12	16	18	17	16
008	Grand Rapids Comm College Mrs Marilyn Smidt, Dir *Chair's #: (616) 771-4231*	143 Bostwick, NE Grand Rapids	49502			A	CC	PBL	10	12	110	109	44	36
016	Grand Rapids Educ Center Ms Suzette Buha, Coord *Chair's #: (616) 364-8464*	1750 Woolworth Grand Rapids	49505	1			TCH	PBL			Publication withheld			
005	Great Lakes Jr College Mrs Barbara Carter, Dir *Chair's #: (517) 835-4501*	3555 East Patrick Rd Midland	48642	7			CC	PVT			Data reported w/AD prog			

Explanation of footnotes on page x

School Code	Name of School, Director of Program, and Phone Number	Street Address / City or Town and Zip Code		Footnotes	Type of Program	NLNAC Accreditation as of January 31, 1998	Administrative Control	Financial Support (principal source)	Number of Months in Program	Educational Requirements for Entering Adult Program	Enrollments as of October 15, 1997	Admissions Aug. 1, 1996 - July 31, 1997	Graduations Aug. 1, 1996 - July 31, 1997	Fall Admissions Aug. 1, 1997 - Dec. 31, 1997
	MICHIGAN													
	- Continued													
018	Jackson Comm College Ms Kathy Walsh, Chair Chair's #: (517) 787-0800 Ext 8515	2111 Emmons Rd Jackson	49201				CC	PBL	13	12	42	50	0	0
023	JTPA Sch of Practical Nursing Ms Lula Johnson, Acting Dir Chair's #: (313) 596-7608	735 Griswold Detroit	48226			A	SEC	PBL	12	12	98	119	83	59
044	Kalamazoo Valley Comm College Mrs Carol Roe, Director Chair's #: (616) 372-5365	6767 West O Ave Kalamazoo	49009	7			CC	PBL			Data reported w/AD prog			
006	Kellogg Comm College Mrs Cynthia Sublett, Dir Chair's #: (616) 965-3931 Ext 2309	450 North Ave Battle Creek	49016				CC	PBL			22	22	19	27
043	Kirtland Comm College Ms Maryann Fleischmann, Chair Chair's #: (517) 275-5121 Ext 298	10775 N St Helen Rd Roscommon	48653				CC	PBL	9	12	46	50	36	50
020	Lake Michigan College Mrs Alice Rasmussen, Coord Chair's #: (616) 927-8100 Ext 5092	2755 E Napier Ave Benton Harbor	49022	7			CC	PBL			Data reported w/AD Prog			
004	Lansing Comm College Ms Dorothy Linau-Mirkil, Coord Chair's #: (517) 483-1410	419 N Capitol Ave Lansing	48914	7			CC	PBL			Data reported w/AD Prog			
037	Mid-Michigan Comm College Mrs Beth Sendre, Director Chair's #: (517) 386-6645	1375 S Clare Ave Harrison	48625	7			CC	PBL			Data reported w/AD Prog			
035	Montcalm Comm College Ms Catherine Earl, Director Chair's #: (517) 328-1240	Sidney	48885				CC	PBL			Publication withheld			
021	Muskegon County Comm College Mrs Darlene Collet, Director Chair's #: (616) 777-0332	221 S Quarterline Rd Muskegon	49443	7			CC	PBL			Data Reported w/AD Prog			
009	Northern Michigan Univ-PN Dept Ms Cheryl Karvonen, Dept Head Chair's #: (906) 227-2640	College Of Nursing Marquette	49855				COL	PBL			Publication withheld			
010	NW Michigan College-PN Ctr Mrs Ann Cook, Coord Chair's #: (616) 922-1238	1701 E Front St Traverse City	49684				CC	PBL	12	12	34	27	13	20
025	Oakland Comm College Ms Karon Schartz, Dean Chair's #: (248) 360-6240	7350 Cooley Lake Rd Waterford	48327				CC	PBL	12	12	25	33	19	25

School Code	Name of School, Director of Program, and Phone Number	Street Address, City or Town and Zip Code		Footnotes	Type of Program	NLNAC Accreditation as of January 31, 1998	Administrative Control	Financial Support (principal source)	Number of Months in Program	Educational Requirements for Entering Adult Program	Enrollments as of October 15, 1997	Admissions Aug. 1, 1996 - July 31, 1997	Graduations Aug. 1, 1996 - July 31, 1997	Fall Admissions Aug. 1, 1997 - Dec. 31, 1997
	MICHIGAN													
	- Continued													
027	Schoolcraft College Mrs Midge Carleton, Asst Dean Chair's #: (734) 462-4400 Ext 5226	18600 Haggerty Rd Livonia	48151				CC	PBL			Publication withheld			
034	Southwestern Michigan Coll Miss Marilouise Hagenberg, Dean Chair's #: (616) 782-1237	58900 Cherry Grove Rd Dowagiac	49047	7			CC	PBL			Data reported w/AD prog			
015	St Clair Co Comm College Mrs Susan J Meeker, Dir Chair's #: (810) 989-5680	323 Erie St PO Box 5015 Port Huron	48061				CC	PBL	12	12	125	82	96	39
038	West Shore Comm College Mrs Patricia Collins, Dir Chair's #: (616) 845-6211 Ext 3518	PO Box 277 Scottville	49454				CC	PBL	11	12	28	30	24	30
	MINNESOTA													
	26 Programs in 26 Schools													
024	Alexandria Tech College Mrs Jola Amundsen, Director Chair's #: (320) 762-4447	1601 Jefferson St Alexandria	56308				TCH	PBL	11	12	62	64	57	32
032	Anoka-Hennepin Tech College Ms Glenda Jensen, Dir Chair's #: (612) 576-4959	1355 W Hwy 10 Anoka	55303			A	TCH	PBL	0	12	101	103	63	24
018	Central Lake College Mrs Genevieve Holden, Dir Chair's #: (218) 828-2525	501W College Dr Brainerd	56401				COL	PBL			Publication withheld			
040	Dakota County Tech College-PN Prog Ms Meri Beth Kennedy, Dir Chair's #: (612) 423-8000 Ext 311	1300 145th St East Rosemount	55068	HSE		A A	TCH TCH	PBL PBL	12	12 12	208 0	78 0	82 0	108 0
027	Fergus Falls Comm College Mrs Donna Quam, Coord Chair's #: (218) 739-7500 Ext 7546	1414 College Way Fergus Falls	56537				CC	PBL	9	12	25	31	24	30
039	Hennepin Tech College Ms Anne Cassens, Dir Chair's #: (612) 550-3166	9200 Flying Cloud Dr Eden Prairie	55347				TCH	PBL			Publication withheld			
026	Itasca Comm College Ms Charlene Sawyer, Director Chair's #: (218) 327-4469	1851 Hwy 169 E Grand Rapids	55744				CC	PBL	10	12	30	37	24	31
002	Lake Superior Coll Ms Carleen Ronchetti, Dir Chair's #: (218) 733-7635	2101 Trinity Rd Duluth	55811				TCH	PBL	15	12	270	246	58	270

Explanation of footnotes on page x

School Code	Name of School, Director of Program, and Phone Number	Street Address / City or Town and Zip Code		Footnotes	Type of Program	NLNAC Accreditation as of January 31, 1998	Administrative Control	Financial Support (principal source)	Number of Months in Program	Educational Requirements for Entering Adult Program	Enrollments as of October 15, 1997	Admissions Aug. 1, 1996 - July 31, 1997	Graduations Aug. 1, 1996 - July 31, 1997	Fall Admissions Aug. 1, 1997 - Dec. 31, 1997
	MINNESOTA													
	- Continued													
035	Mesabi Range Tech College PN Prog Mrs Mary Zahorsky, Director *Chair's #: (218) 744-7456*	1100 Industrial Pk Dr Eveleth	55734				TCH	PBL	15	12	34	32	29	32
006	Minneapolis Comm Tech Coll Dr Joanne M Wandrei, Dean *Chair's #: (612) 359-1363*	1501 Hennepin Ave So Minneapolis	55403			A	CC	PBL	15	12	190	156	71	61
044	Minnesota West Comm And Tech Coll Mrs Jacqueline Otkin, Director *Chair's #: (507) 825-4054 Ext 237*	Box 250 Pipestone	56164				TCH	PBL	12	12	38	38	19	38
037	Minnesota West Comm and Tech Coll Ms Kathi Haberman, Dir *Chair's #: (507) 372-3443 Ext 3443*	1450 Collegeway Worthington	56187				CC	PBL	13	12	25	30	19	0
013	Northland Comm And Tech Coll Ms Debra Filer, Dean *Chair's #: (218) 681-0841*	1101 Hwy One E Thief River Falls	56701		HS HSE	CC CC CC	PBL PBL PBL	15 15 15	12 12 12	143 4	75 3	31 0	68 4
031	Northwest Tech Coll Ms Ruthann Yliniemi, Dir *Chair's #: (218) 847-1341 Ext 316*	900 Highway 34 E Detroit Lakes	56501				TCH	PBL			Publication withheld			
029	Northwest Tech Coll Mrs Karen Sollom, Director *Chair's #: (218) 755-4270*	905 Grant Ave SE Bemidji	56601				TCH	PBL			Publication withheld			
038	Northwest Tech College Ms Mary Wiersma, Dir *Chair's #: (218) 773-4556*	Highway 220 N East Grand Forks	56721				TCH	PBL			40	50	30	20
042	Rainy River Comm Coll-PN Prog Mrs Judy Junker, Director *Chair's #: (218) 285-7722*	1501 Highway 71 Internatl Falls	56649				CC	PBL			33	40	15	33
012	Red Wing-Winona Campus Ms Laurie Becker, Director *Chair's #: (507) 453-2635*	110 Galewski Dr Winona	55987		HSE		TCH TCH	PBL PBL	12	12 12	105 0	152 0	39 0	58 0
014	Red Wing-Winona Tech Coll Ms Marsha Edblom Zich, Dir *Chair's #: (612) 385-6300 Ext 6371*	308 Pioneer Rd Red Wing	55066		HSE		TCH TCH	PBL PBL	11	12 12	74 0	109 0	28 0	31 0
011	Ridgewater College Mrs Janet Jaeger, Director *Chair's #: (320) 231-2950*	2101 15th Ave NW Box 1097 Willmar	56201			A	TCH	PBL	12	12	107	106	64	71
004	Riverland Comm Coll Ms Patricia Parson, Dir *Chair's #: (507) 453-0826*	1900 Eighth Ave NW Austin	55912				CC	PBL	15	12	16	53	20	39

School Code	Name of School, Director of Program, and Phone Number	Street Address / City or Town and Zip Code		Footnotes	Type of Program	NLNAC Accreditation as of January 31, 1998	Administrative Control	Financial Support (principal source)	Number of Months in Program	Educational Requirements for Entering Adult Program	Enrollments as of October 15, 1997	Admissions Aug. 1, 1996 - July 31, 1997	Graduations Aug. 1, 1996 - July 31, 1997	Fall Admissions Aug. 1, 1997 - Dec. 31, 1997
	MINNESOTA													
	- Continued													
015	Rochester Comm And Tech Coll Ms Lorna Schmidt, Dir *Chair's #: (507) 280-3161*	851 30th Ave SE Rochester	55904			A	TCH	PBL			Publication withheld			
034	South Central Tech Coll Mrs Phyllis Wegner, Dir *Chair's #: (507) 389-7200*	1920 Lee Blvd N Mankato	56002				TCH	PBL			Publication withheld			
005	South Central Tech Coll Ms Phyllis Wegner, Dir *Chair's #: (507) 332-5801*	1225 Third St SW Faribault	55021				TCH	PBL	12	12	73	59	40	37
030	St Cloud Tech College PN Prog Mrs Renea Barclay, Dir *Chair's #: (320) 255-3700*	1540 Northway Dr St Cloud	56303			A	TCH	PBL	15	12	117	80	65	26
036	St Paul Tech College PN Prog Dr Marilyn Krasowski, Dir *Chair's #: (612) 221-1314*	235 Marshall Ave St Paul	55102			A	TCH	PBL	12	12	151	213	56	123
	MISSISSIPPI													
	16 Programs in 15 Schools													
900	Coahoma Comm Coll Mr Jerone Shaw, Coord *Chair's #: (601) 627-2571 Ext 291*	3240 Friars Pt Rd Clarksdale	38614				CC	PBL			Publication withheld			
047	Copiah-Lincoln Comm College (2 Brchs Mr Louis Dugas, Dean *Chair's #: (601) 643-8322*	Wesson	39191				CC	PBL	12	12	25	30	18	28
081	East Central Comm College Mr John Addock, Dir *Chair's #: (601) 635-2111 Ext 211*	PO Box 129 Decatur	39327				CC	PBL			Publication withheld			
050	East MS Comm College Mrs Denise Tennison, Chair *Chair's #: (601) 243-1945*	Golden Triangle Campus-Box 1 May Hew	39753				CC	PVT	11	12	33	46	23	36
012	Hinds Comm College (2 Branches) Ms Sandra Freeman, Chair *Chair's #: (601) 371-3516*	1750 Chadwick Dr Jackson	39204				TCH	PBL			Publication withheld			
046	Holmes Comm College (5 Branches) Mrs Gail Caraway, Director *Chair's #: (601) 472-2820*	Box 369 Goodman	39079				CC	PBL			Publication withheld			
032	Itawamba Comm College Ms Treny Guntharp, Dir *Chair's #: (601) 680-8451 Ext 451*	653 Eason Blvd Tupelo	38801				TCH	PBL			Publication withheld			

Explanation of footnotes on page x

School Code	Name of School, Director of Program, and Phone Number	Street Address, City or Town and Zip Code		Footnotes	Type of Program	NLNAC Accreditation as of January 31, 1998	Administrative Control	Financial Support (principal source)	Number of Months in Program	Educational Requirements for Entering Adult Program	Enrollments as of October 15, 1997	Admissions Aug. 1, 1996 - July 31, 1997	Graduations Aug. 1, 1996 - July 31, 1997	Fall Admissions Aug. 1, 1997 - Dec. 31, 1997
	MISSISSIPPI													
	- Continued													
091	Jones County Junior College Ms Sandra Waldrup, Dir *Chair's #: (601) 477-4101*	Ellisville	39437				CC	PBL	12	12	73	80	73	40
099	Meridian Comm College Ms Rowena Saucier, Coord *Chair's #: (601) 483-8241 Ext 725*	910 Hwy 19 N Meridian	39301			A	CC	PBL	12	12	53	71	44	31
090	Mississippi Delta Comm College (3 Brc Dr Martha Heffner, Asst Dean *Chair's #: (601) 246-6322*	Moorhead	38761				CC	PBL		Publication withheld				
096	MS Gulf Coast Comm College (3 Brchs) Dr Judith Benvenutti, Dir *Chair's #: (601) 928-6335*	PO Box 27 Perkinston	39573				CC	PBL	12	12	91	102	65	104
044	NE Mississippi Comm College Mr Kenneth Pounders, Div Head *Chair's #: (601) 720-7207*	Booneville	38829				CC	PBL	12	12	36	36	25	24
089	NW Mississippi Comm Coll (3 Branche Mr Joe Broadway, Director *Chair's #: (601) 562-3232*	Senatobia	38668				CC	PBL		Publication withheld				
045	Pearl River Comm College (3 Brchs) Ms Edith Royse, Chair *Chair's #: (601) 554-9136*	101 Hwy 11 No-Box 5760 Poplarville	39470				CC	PBL	12	12	52	52	46	53
021	SW Mississippi Comm Coll Mrs Frances Morris, Coord *Chair's #: (601) 276-2000 Ext 3851*	Summit	39666				TCH	PBL		Publication withheld				
	MISSOURI													
	41 Programs in 41 Schools													
016	Applied Technology Services/W County Mrs Maudie Streetman, Coord *Chair's #: (314) 579-4805*	13480 South Outer 40 Hwy Chesterfield	63117				TCH	PBL	12	12	29	36	31	18
044	Boonslick Area Voc-Tech School Mrs Janie Higgins, Coord *Chair's #: (660) 882-5306*	1694 Ashley Rd Boonville	65233				TCH	PVT	12	12	27	20	17	27
043	Cape Girardeau Area Voc-Tech Sch Mrs C Eaker-Kranawetter, Coord *Chair's #: (573) 335-7708 Ext 26*	301 N Clark Cape Girardeau	63701				TCH	PBL	12	12	25	24	18	25
011	Columbia Public Schs-PN Program Mrs Sharon Taylor, Asst Dir *Chair's #: (573) 886-2276*	500 Strawn Rd Columbia	65203			A	TCH	PBL	12	12	60	62	45	32

School Code	Name of School, Director of Program, and Phone Number	Street Address / City or Town and Zip Code		Footnotes	Type of Program	NLNAC Accreditation as of January 31, 1998	Administrative Control	Financial Support (principal source)	Number of Months in Program	Educational Requirements for Entering Adult Program	Enrollments as of October 15, 1997	Admissions Aug. 1, 1996 - July 31, 1997	Graduations Aug. 1, 1996 - July 31, 1997	Fall Admissions Aug. 1, 1997 - Dec. 31, 1997
	MISSOURI													
	- Continued													
046	Gibson AVTS Mrs Joann Chalfant, Coord *Chair's #: (417) 272-3459*	PO Box 169 Reeds Spring	65737				TCH	PBL			32	31	24	34
017	Hannibal Public Sch of PN Mrs Gwenda Pollard, Coord *Chair's #: (573) 221-4430 Ext 182*	4550 McMasters Ave Hannibal	63401				TCH	PVT	12	12	22	24	19	23
036	Jefferson College Ms Michele Soest, Director *Chair's #: (314) 789-3951 Ext 409*	1000 Viking Dr Hillsboro	63050				CC	PBL	10	12	49	45	39	51
041	Kennett AVTS Ms Betty Poindexter, Coord *Chair's #: (573) 717-1123*	1400 W Washington Kennett	63857				TCH	PBL	12	12	18	20	17	21
024	Kirksville ATC Mrs Sherry Willis, Coord *Chair's #: (660) 626-1470*	1103 S Cottage Grove Kirksville	63501				TCH	PBL	12	12	23	25	21	24
032	Lex La-Ray Technical Center Ms Bernice Wagner, Coord *Chair's #: (816) 259-2264 Ext 173*	2323 High School Dr Lexington	64067				TCH	PBL	12	12	22	28	20	25
018	Mineral Area College, The Prog in PN Mrs Lana Harris, Coord *Chair's #: (573) 431-4593 Ext 276*	PO Box 1000 Park Hills	63601				CC	PBL			Publication withheld			
035	Moberly Area Comm Coll Ms Ruth Jones, Dir *Chair's #: (573) 581-1925*	1320 Paris Rd Mexico	65265	1			CC	PBL			Publication withheld			
027	Moberly Area Comm College Ms Terry Bichsel, Coord *Chair's #: (816) 263-4110 Ext 251*	101 College Ave Moberly	65270	7			CC	PBL			Data reported w/AD prog			
021	N S Hillyard Tech Sch Mrs Patricia Alft, Coord *Chair's #: (816) 671-4170 Ext 26*	3434 Faraon St St Joseph	64506				TCH	PBL	11	12	23	25	24	24
023	Nevada Regional Tech Center Ms Rebecca Householder, Coord *Chair's #: (417) 448-2016*	2015 N West St Nevada	64772				TCH	PBL	12	12	25	29	26	24
015	Nichols Career Ctr Mrs Patricia Francka, Coord *Chair's #: (573) 659-3111*	609 Union St Jefferson City	65101			A	TCH	PBL	12	12	32	34	26	34
020	North Central MO College Ms Pat Dixon, Assoc Dean *Chair's #: (660) 359-3948 Ext 310*	1301 E Main St Trenton	64683	7			CC	PBL			Data reported w/AD prog			

Explanation of footnotes on page x

School Code	Name of School, Director of Program, and Phone Number	Street Address / City or Town and Zip Code		Footnotes	Type of Program	NLNAC Accreditation as of January 31, 1998	Administrative Control	Financial Support (principal source)	Number of Months in Program	Educational Requirements for Entering Adult Program	Enrollments as of October 15, 1997	Admissions Aug. 1, 1996 - July 31, 1997	Graduations Aug. 1, 1996 - July 31, 1997	Fall Admissions Aug. 1, 1997 - Dec. 31, 1997
	MISSOURI - Continued													
049	Northland Career Ctr AVTS Mrs Betty Boles, Coord *Chair's #: (816) 858-5505 Ext 21*	PO Box 1700 Platte City	64079				TCH	PBL	13	12	28	28	23	28
031	Northwest Technical Sch Ms Trudith S Dorrel, Coord *Chair's #: (660) 562-3022 Ext 4139*	1515 South Munn Maryville	64468				TCH	PBL	11	12	25	25	22	25
012	Ozarks Tech Comm Coll Mrs Sandra Richarson, Dean *Chair's #: (417) 895-7135*	PO Box 5958 Springfield	65801				CC	PBL	10	12	34	49	58	18
003	Penn Valley Comm College Ms Alice Wilson, Coord *Chair's #: (816) 482-5070*	2700 E 18th St Kansas City	64127			A	CC	PBL	12	12	35	76	58	24
042	Pike/Lincoln Tech Center Mrs Gail Branstetter, Coord *Chair's #: (573) 485-2900 Ext 11*	Rt 1A Box 38 Eolia	63344				TCH	PBL	12	12	10	23	13	12
007	Poplar Bluff Sch Dist, PN Prog Ms Jana Scott, Coord *Chair's #: (573) 785-6867*	PO Box 47 Poplar Bluff	63902				TCH	PBL			Publication withheld			
026	Rolla Tech Inst Mrs Pati Cox, Coord *Chair's #: (573) 364-3726 Ext 130*	1304 E 10th St Rolla	65401				TCH	PBL	12	12	31	31	26	31
030	Saline Co Career Center Mrs Stefanie Sauble, Admin *Chair's #: (660) 886-6958*	900 W Vest Marshall	65340				TCH	PBL			Publication withheld			
901	Sanford Brown Coll Ms Vickie Baker-Janis, Dir *Chair's #: (314) 949-2620*	3555 Franks Dr St Charles	63301				TCH	PVT			See N Kansas City Campus			
900	Sanford Brown Coll Ms Sheryl Zysk, Coord *Chair's #: (314) 822-7100*	12006 Manchester Rd St Louis	63131				TCH	PVT			See N Kansas City Campus			
008	Sanford Brown Coll Ms Cheryl Hendricks Scott, Dir *Chair's #: (816) 472-7400*	520 E 19th Ave N Kansas City	64116				TCH	PVT			126	153	139	51
010	School Dist of Joplin R-VIII Ms Joyce Stevenson, Coord *Chair's #: (417) 659-4403*	3950 East Newman Joplin	64804				TCH	PBL	12	12	48	54	39	27
022	Sikeston Public Schs (2 Branches) Mrs Pat Elledge, Coord *Chair's #: (573) 472-8887*	1002 Virginia Sikeston	63801			A	TCH	PBL	11	12	42	51	46	0

Explanation of footnotes on page x

School Code	Name of School, Director of Program, and Phone Number	Street Address City or Town and Zip Code		Footnotes	Type of Program	NLNAC Accreditation as of January 31, 1998	Administrative Control	Financial Support (principal source)	Number of Months in Program	Educational Requirements for Entering Adult Program	Enrollments as of October 15, 1997	Admissions Aug. 1, 1996 - July 31, 1997	Graduations Aug. 1, 1996 - July 31, 1997	Fall Admissions Aug. 1, 1997 - Dec. 31, 1997
	MISSOURI													
	- Continued													
033	South Central AVTS Ms Marlene Martensen, Admin *Chair's #: (417) 256-6150 Ext 212*	613 W First St West Plains	65775				TCH	PBL	12	12	28	30	25	28
048	St Charles Co Comm College Ms Russlyn St John, Coord *Chair's #: (314) 922-8280*	4601 Mid River Mall Dr St Peters	63376				CC	PBL	14	12	14	13	17	0
002	St Louis Bd of Education PN Ms Mitzi Bryant, Coord *Chair's #: (314) 781-1322 Ext 250*	3815 McCausland Ave St Louis	63109				TCH	PBL	12	12	54	33	49	22
050	St Louis Coll of Hlth Career Mrs Deborah Goldseder, Dir *Chair's #: (314) 652-0300*	4484 West Pine Blvd St Louis	63108				TCH	PVT			Publication withheld			
006	St Louis Coll of Hlth Career Mrs Deborah Goldseder, Dir *Chair's #: (314) 845-6100*	4044 Butler Hill Rd St Louis	63129	1			TCH	PVT			Publication withheld			
028	State Fair Comm College Ms Leora Bremer, Coord *Chair's #: (816) 530-5800 Ext 228*	3201 W 16th St Sedalia	65301				CC	PBL	10	12	30	34	32	30
004	Tri County Tech Sch Mrs Susan Green, Coord *Chair's #: (573) 392-8060*	2nd & Pine St Eldon	65026				TCH	PVT	12	12	25	25	17	0
038	Warrensburg AVTS Mrs Marcile R Lewis, Coord *Chair's #: (660) 747-2283*	205 S Ridgeview Dr Warrensburg	64093				TCH	PBL	12		28	28	21	30
034	Washington School of PN Mrs Christie Gildehaus, Coord *Chair's #: (314) 239-7777*	550 East Eleventh St Washington	63090				TCH	PBL	11	12	21	27	21	24
040	Waynesville Tech Academy Mrs Glenda Cole, Coord *Chair's #: (573) 774-6584*	810 Roosevelt St Waynesville	65583				TCH	PBL	12	12	29	30	23	30
	MONTANA													
	5 Programs in 5 Schools													
010	Helena College of Technology Ms Patricia A Herold, Coord *Chair's #: (406) 444-6800 Ext 1226*	2300 Poplar St Helena	59601				TCH	PBL			Publication withheld			
011	Montana State Univ-Billings Voc-Tech Dr Audrey Conner Rosberg, Dir *Chair's #: (406) 656-4445 Ext 150*	3803 Central Ave Billings	59102				TCH	PBL	24	12	98	67	32	44

Explanation of footnotes on page x

School Code	Name of School, Director of Program, and Phone Number	Street Address, City or Town and Zip Code	Footnotes	Type of Program	NLNAC Accreditation as of January 31, 1998	Administrative Control	Financial Support (principal source)	Number of Months in Program	Educational Requirements for Entering Adult Program	Enrollments as of October 15, 1997	Admissions Aug. 1, 1996 - July 31, 1997	Graduations Aug. 1, 1996 - July 31, 1997	Fall Admissions Aug. 1, 1997 - Dec. 31, 1997
	MONTANA												
	- Continued												
012	Montana Tech/Coll of Technology Mrs Karen Vandaveer, Director *Chair's #: (406) 496-3722*	Basin Creek Rd Butte 59701				TCH	PBL	12	12	48	38	28	18
004	MSU College of Technology Ms Connie MacKay, Dir *Chair's #: (406) 771-4352*	2100 16th Ave South Great Falls 59405				TCH	PBL	12	12	10	50	28	10
003	Univ of Montana Coll of Tech Ms Margaret A Wafstet, Dir *Chair's #: (406) 243-7864*	909 South Ave, W Missoula 59801				CC	PBL	16	12	69	58	38	28
	NEBRASKA												
	8 Programs in 8 Schools												
006	Central Comm College (3 Branches) Mrs Linda Walline, Assoc Dean *Chair's #: (308) 389-6456*	PO Box 4903 3134 W Hwy 34 Grand Island 68502				TCH	PBL	11	12	82	99	65	63
001	Metropolitan Comm College Dr Janice T Adkins, Chair *Chair's #: (402) 457-2367*	PO Box 3777 Omaha 68103				CC	PBL	15	12	25	30	26	30
008	Mid-Plains Comm College Mrs Pauline Shahan, Dept Head *Chair's #: (308) 532-8740 Ext 252*	1101 Hallgan Dr North Platte 69101			A	CC	PBL	12	12	42	43	30	35
005	Northeast Comm College Mrs Anita Brenneman, Chair *Chair's #: (402) 644-0444 Ext 4444*	801 E Benjamin Ave PO Box 4 Norfolk 68702				CC	PBL	12	12	34	53	38	22
004	SE Nebraska Comm College-Lincoln Ms Iris Winkelhake, Chair *Chair's #: (402) 437-2765*	8800 O St Lincoln 68520			A	CC	PBL	12	12	56	58	49	28
009	Southeast Comm College-Beatrice Cam Mrs Crystal Higgins, Chair *Chair's #: (402) 228-3469 Ext 264*	PO Box 35A Beatrice 68310			A	CC	PBL	12	12	47	58	35	9
003	Western Nebraska Comm College (2 Brc Ms Anne Hippe, Chair *Chair's #: (308) 635-6181*	1601 East 35th Scottsbluff 69361			A	CC	PBL	0	12	39	30	24	39
	NEVADA												
	1 Program in 1 School												
010	W Nevada Comm College-Carson City Ms Mildred Wade, Dir *Chair's #: (702) 887-3176*	2201 W College Parkway Carson City 89701	7			CC	PBL			Data reported w/AD Prog			

School Code	Name of School, Director of Program, and Phone Number	Street Address / City or Town and Zip Code	Footnotes	Type of Program	NLNAC Accreditation as of January 31, 1998	Administrative Control	Financial Support (principal source)	Number of Months in Program	Educational Requirements for Entering Adult Program	Enrollments as of October 15, 1997	Admissions Aug. 1, 1996 - July 31, 1997	Graduations Aug. 1, 1996 - July 31, 1997	Fall Admissions Aug. 1, 1997 - Dec. 31, 1997
	NEW HAMPSHIRE												
	4 Programs in 2 Schools												
006	New Hampshire Tech College-Claremon Dr Susan Henderson, Chair Chair's #: (603) 542-7744 Ext 39	One College Dr RR#3 Box 550 Claremont 03743				CC	PBL	11		40	48	34	40
004	St Joseph Sch of Practical Nsg Dr Judith Haywood, Dir Chair's #: (603) 888-1311 Ext 8530	5 Woodward Ave Nashua 03060			A	HSP	PVT	11		105	62	68	49
	NEW JERSEY												
	23 Programs in 23 Schools												
029	Atlantic County Voc Sch Ms Rosalie G Mocco, Coord Chair's #: (609) 625-2249 Ext 1315	5080 Atlantic Ave Mays Landing 08330				TCH	PBL	12	12	27	32	27	32
009	Bergen Pines County Hosp Mrs Joanne Frazer, Asst Dir Chair's #: (201) 967-4088	E Ridgewood Ave Paramus 07652			A	HSP	PBL	12	12	21	79	46	0
022	Burlington Co Voc and Tech Schs Mrs Alice Sinclair, Supv Chair's #: (609) 654-0200 Ext 426	Medford Campus Hawkins Rd Medford 08055				TCH	PBL	11	12	33	60	47	33
027	Camden Bd of Education Ms Danna Beverly, Coord Chair's #: (609) 966-2479	1656 Kaighns Ave Camden 08103				SEC	PBL	18	12	42	26	16	26
004	Camden Co Voc Tech Sch Mrs Flax E Brooks, Coord Chair's #: (609) 767-7000 Ext 5540	343 Berlin Cross Keys Rd Sicklerville 08081				TCH	PBL	12	12	18	22	15	21
021	Cape May Co Tech Inst Mr Rusty Miller, Supv Chair's #: (609) 465-2161 Ext 645	Crest Haven Rd Cape May C H 08210				TCH	PBL	11	12	20	22	13	22
035	Cumberland County Tech Educ Center Mrs Priscilla Meyers, Coord Chair's #: (609) 451-9000 Ext 245	601 Bridgeton Ave Bridgeton 08302				TCH	PBL	12	12	21	34	26	22
001	Essex Co Tech Careers Ctr Mrs Loraine San Roman, Coord Chair's #: (973) 622-1100 Ext 349	91 W Market St Newark 07103				TCH	PBL	12	12	29	28	48	31
044	Gloucester Co Voc School Ms Patricia A Mulutzie, Coord Chair's #: (609) 875-3600	PO Box 800 Tanyard Rd Sewell 08080				TCH	PBL			Publication withheld			
038	Holy Name Hosp Sr Claire Tynan, Senior Vice Pres Chair's #: (201) 833-3008	690 Teaneck Rd Teaneck 07666				HSP	PVT	12	12	30	33	25	30

Explanation of footnotes on page x

School Code	Name of School, Director of Program, and Phone Number	Street Address City or Town and Zip Code		Footnotes	Type of Program	NLNAC Accreditation as of January 31, 1998	Administrative Control	Financial Support (principal source)	Number of Months in Program	Educational Requirements for Entering Adult Program	Enrollments as of October 15, 1997	Admissions Aug. 1, 1996 - July 31, 1997	Graduations Aug. 1, 1996 - July 31, 1997	Fall Admissions Aug. 1, 1997 - Dec. 31, 1997
	NEW JERSEY													
	- Continued													
026	Hudson County Voc Sch Mrs Carol Cruden, Dir *Chair's #: (201) 339-1673*	W 30th St Bayonne	07002				TCH	PBL			Publication withheld			
034	Mercer County Voc Sch-HOC Mrs V Clevenger, Supv *Chair's #: (609) 587-7640*	1070 Klockner Rd Trenton	08619				TCH	PBL	12	12	48	35	32	42
039	Middlesex Co V-T Sch of PN (4 Brchs) Mrs Joan McNulty, Director *Chair's #: (732) 613-9201*	112 Rues Ln Box 220 East Brunswick	08816				TCH	PBL			Publication withheld			
015	Monmouth County Voc Sch Dist Mrs Iris Arbeitman, Dir *Chair's #: (732) 229-7676*	185 State Route 36 West Long Branch	07764				TCH	PBL	12	10	134	115	103	60
037	Morris Co Voc Sch Mr Gene Polles, Director *Chair's #: (201) 627-4600 Ext 232*	400 E Main St Denville	07834				TCH	PBL			Publication withheld			
016	Ocean County Voc Tech Sch Mrs Barbara Haines, Vice Principal *Chair's #: (732) 473-3139*	1299 Old Freehold Rd Toms River	08753				TCH	PBL	11	12	76	101	42	42
007	Passaic Co Tech And Voc Hs Ms Athena Fitzgerald, Coord *Chair's #: (973) 628-9208*	1006 Hamburg Turnpike Wayne	07470				SEC	PBL			Publication withheld			
013	Salem Comm College Mrs Louise Murphy, Dir *Chair's #: (609) 351-2648*	Carneys Point	08069				CC	PBL			Publication withheld			
018	Somerset Co Voc-Tech Sch Mrs Louise S McLinden, Supv *Chair's #: (908) 526-8900 Ext 235*	PO Box 6350 Bridgewater	08807				TCH	PBL			Publication withheld			
019	Sussex County Voc-Tech Schs Mrs Maureen S Howard, Dir *Chair's #: (973) 383-6700 Ext 222*	105 North Church Rd Sparta	07871				TCH	PBL	12	12	20	31	24	31
023	Union County College Miss Ellen Boddie, Dir *Chair's #: (908) 965-6088 Ext 6088*	12-24 W Jersey St Elizabeth	07202		A		CC	PBL	12	12	180	128	156	0
028	Vineland Adult Center Mrs Gloria Rochetti, Director *Chair's #: (609) 794-6943*	48 Landis Ave Vineland	08360				SEC	PBL			Publication withheld			
020	Warren Co Voc Sch and Tech Inst Mr Frank Mancuso, Dir *Chair's #: (908) 689-0122 Ext 14*	Rd 1, Box 168A Washington	07882				TCH	PBL			Publication withheld			

Explanation of footnotes on page x

School Code	Name of School, Director of Program, and Phone Number	Street Address / City or Town and Zip Code	Footnotes	Type of Program	NLNAC Accreditation as of January 31, 1998	Administrative Control	Financial Support (principal source)	Number of Months in Program	Educational Requirements for Entering Adult Program	Enrollments as of October 15, 1997	Admissions Aug. 1, 1996 - July 31, 1997	Graduations Aug. 1, 1996 - July 31, 1997	Fall Admissions Aug. 1, 1997 - Dec. 31, 1997
	NEW MEXICO												
	8 Programs in 8 Schools												
020	Albuquerque Public Schs of PN Mrs Nina Adkins, Chair *Chair's #: (505) 247-3658 Ext 33*	807 Mountain Rd NE Albuquerque 87102	HS		A A	SEC SEC	PBL PBL	20	10	0 68	0 75	0 22	0 74
004	Albuquerque TVI Miss Patricia Stephens, Director *Chair's #: (505) 224-4141*	200 Coal SE Albuquerque 87106			A	CC	PBL	12	12	27	32	25	0
017	Clovis Comm Coll Mrs Ione Wood, Director *Chair's #: (505) 769-4975*	417 Schepps Blvd Clovis 88101				CC	PBL	8	12	39	80	55	40
010	Eastern New Mexico Univ at Roswell Mrs Eloise A Blake, Chair *Chair's #: (505) 624-7235*	PO Box 6000 Roswell 88201	7			CC	PBL	12	12	0	0	8	0
014	Luna Voc Tech Inst Ms Beatrice Hurtado, Interim Dir *Chair's #: (505) 454-2524*	PO Box 1510 Las Vegas 87701				CC	PBL	9	12	22	24	21	22
009	New Mexico Jr College Mr Steven M Davis, Director *Chair's #: (505) 392-5714*	5317 Lovington Highway Hobbs 88240	7			CC	PBL			Data reported w/AD prog			
018	New Mexico State Univ Ms Sharon Souter, Dir *Chair's #: (505) 234-9301*	1500 University Dr Carlsbad 88220	7			CC	PBL			Data reported w/AD prog			
002	Northern New Mexico Comm College Ms Ramona Gonzales, Dir *Chair's #: (505) 747-2209*	1002 N Onate Espanola 87532	7			CC	PBL			Data reported w/AD Prog			
	NEW YORK												
	124 Programs in 54 Schools												
011	Albany-Schoharie-Schenectady BOCES Ms Joanne O'Brien, Coord *Chair's #: (518) 456-9202*	1015 Watervliet-Shaker Rd Albany 12205				TCH	PVT			Publication withheld			
902	Bronx Comm College Mrs Ellen R Hoist, Director *Chair's #: (718) 289-5420*	181 St University Ave Rm 408 Bronx 10453				CC	PVT	18		70	43	27	25
764	Broome-Tioga BOCES Mrs Annette Gould, Coord *Chair's #: (607) 786-8502*	435 Upper Glenwood Rd Binghamton 13905				SEC	PBL	20	12	35	19	15	22
016	Buffalo Voc-Tech Ctr Mrs Kathleen Sorrentino, Admin *Chair's #: (716) 897-8108*	820 Northampton St Buffalo 14211	HSE			GOV GOV	PBL PBL	12 24	12 12	49 6	51 13	34 5	25 6

Explanation of footnotes on page x

School Code	Name of School, Director of Program, and Phone Number	Street Address / City or Town and Zip Code	Footnotes	Type of Program	NLNAC Accreditation as of January 31, 1998	Administrative Control	Financial Support (principal source)	Number of Months in Program	Educational Requirements for Entering Adult Program	Enrollments as of October 15, 1997	Admissions Aug. 1, 1996 - July 31, 1997	Graduations Aug. 1, 1996 - July 31, 1997	Fall Admissions Aug. 1, 1997 - Dec. 31, 1997
	NEW YORK												
	- Continued												
762	Catragus-Allgny-Wyomg-Erie BOCES Mrs Judith Barillo, Specialist *Chair's #: (716) 372-8293 Ext 217*	Windfall Rd, Box 424B Olean 14760				TCH	PBL	12	12	66	53	30	29
				HS		TCH	PBL	21	12	22	16	5	17
				HSE		TCH	PBL		12				
714	Cayuga/Onondaga BOCES Miss Patricia Kenny, Coord *Chair's #: (315) 253-0361 Ext 153*	5980 S St Rd Auburn 13021				TCH	PBL	21		34	22	22	14
				HSE		TCH	PBL	17		15	16	2	20
098	Champlain Valley Tech Educ Center Mrs Joan Rice, Coord *Chair's #: (518) 561-0100 Ext 248*	PO Box 455 Plattsburgh 12901				TCH	PBL			Publication withheld			
064	Clara Barton HS for Hlth Profs Mrs Julia Blair, Dir *Chair's #: (718) 636-4900 Ext 263*	901 Classon Ave Brooklyn 11225				SEC	PBL			0	0	0	0
				HS		SEC	PBL	22		51	39	18	25
091	Curtis HS-Secondary Prog Mrs Lynn Davis, Coord *Chair's #: (718) 273-7380 Ext 305*	105 Hamilton Ave Staten Island 10301				SEC	PBL			0	0	0	0
				HSE		SEC	PBL	22		56	23	17	32
027	Delaware Chen Mad BOCES Mrs Ann Marie Sullivan, Coord *Chair's #: (607) 335-1303 Ext 1303*	Rd # 3 PO Box 307 Norwich 13815				SEC	PBL	10	12	34	18	13	34
742	Delhi Coll of Tech Ms Mary J Giarrusso, Dir *Chair's #: (607) 746-4130*	Delhi 13753				CC	PBL			Publication withheld			
715	Dutchess BOCES Mrs Margaret Muraca, Coord *Chair's #: (914) 486-8045*	Rd 1 Box 369A Salt Pt Turnpik Poughkeepsie 12601				TCH	PBL			Publication withheld			
093	Eastern Suffolk Sch for PN Mrs Carol Powell, Administrator *Chair's #: (516) 286-6592*	350 Martha Ave Bellport 11713			A	TCH	PBL	18	12	125	145	113	125
				IISE	A	TCH	PBL	18	12	74	38	32	74
744	Ed Opportunity Ctr, PN Prog Mrs Margaret Walker, Admin *Chair's #: (716) 546-8660 Ext 234*	305 Andrews St Rochester 14604				TCH	PBL	11	12	55	120	48	60
771	Erie 2 Cattaraugus, BOCES Mrs Marie Beckstrom, Coord *Chair's #: (716) 549-4454*	1020 Central Ave Dunkirk 14048				TCH	PVT	10	12	58	70	53	70
044	Erie BOCES-First Supv Dist Mrs Georgiann Dudek, Coord *Chair's #: (716) 821-7033*	355 Harlem Rd West Seneca 14224				TCH	PBL	10	12	77	88	108	40
				HSE		TCH	PBL	16	12	82	106	0	82
003	Genesse Livingston Steuben Ms Carolyn Thomas, Coord *Chair's #: (716) 344-7788*	8250 State Street Rd Batavia 14020				TCH	PBL	10	12	36	43	25	43

School Code	Name of School, Director of Program, and Phone Number	Street Address, City or Town and Zip Code		Footnotes	Type of Program	NLNAC Accreditation as of January 31, 1998	Administrative Control	Financial Support (principal source)	Number of Months in Program	Educational Requirements for Entering Adult Program	Enrollments as of October 15, 1997	Admissions Aug. 1, 1996 - July 31, 1997	Graduations Aug. 1, 1996 - July 31, 1997	Fall Admissions Aug. 1, 1997 - Dec. 31, 1997
	NEW YORK													
	- Continued													
710	Hamilton-Fulton Montgmry BOCES Mrs Judith Gisondi, Coord *Chair's #: (518) 762-4633 Ext 124*	212 Co Hwy 103 Box 665 Johnstown	12095		HS		SEC SEC	PBL PBL	21 21	12 12	9 8	22 4	10 1	12 8
705	Herkimer BOCES Ms Karolyn Lado, Coord *Chair's #: (315) 867-2040*	Gros Blvd E Herkimer	13350				TCH	PBL	11	12	53	51	35	41
745	Hillcrest HS Mrs L Dunworth, Asst Principal *Chair's #: (718) 658-5407 Ext 362*	160-05 Highland Ave Jamaica	11432		HSE		SEC SEC	PBL PBL	21		0 76	0 32	0 15	0 64
768	Iona College Mrs Catherine D'Amico, Dir *Chair's #: (914) 633-2129*	715 North Ave New Rochelle	10801			A	COL	PVT			102	102	70	96
069	Isabella G Hart Sch-Rochester Gen Hosp Mrs Nina Morris, Dir *Chair's #: (716) 338-4784*	1425 Portland Ave Rochester	14621		HS	A A	HSP HSP	PVT PVT			Publication withheld			
094	Jefferson-Lewis Co BOCES Prog Mrs Diane Riddell, Coord *Chair's #: (315) 788-3410 Ext 308*	Arsenal St, Rd 1 Watertown	13601		HS		TCH TCH	PBL PBL	11 22		64 45	51 41	59 19	38 45
718	Madison & Oneida BOCES PN Prog Ms Bonnie Servage, Coord *Chair's #: (315) 361-5800*	Spring Rd Verona	13478		HS		SEC SEC	PBL PBL	10 22	10 10	57 17	77 13	53 11	60 17
017	Marion S Whelan Sch of Practical Nsg Ms E Ann McGuane, Director *Chair's #: (315) 787-4003*	196-198 North St Geneva	14456			A	HSP	PVT	12		14	22	17	22
008	Medgar Evers Coll of CUNY Ms Delores Casey, Coord *Chair's #: (212) 270-6442*	1650 Bedford Ave Brooklyn	11222				COL	PBL			Publication withheld			
738	Nassau BOCES Mrs Eileen Brown, Coord *Chair's #: (516) 622-6901*	1196 Prospect Ave Westbury	11590		HS	A A	TCH TCH	PBL PBL	11 20		295 79	221 63	240 31	160 41
770	New York City Bd Educ (2 Branches) Ms Linda Armstrong, Coord *Chair's #: (212) 666-2116*	212 W 120th St Rm 307A New York	10007				TCH	PBL			Publication withheld			
900	Niagara Co Comm College-Nsg Educ Mrs Catherine Peuquet, Director *Chair's #: (716) 731-3271 Ext 267*	3111 Saunders Settlement Rd Sanborn	14132				CC	PBL			Publication withheld			
724	North Country Comm College Mrs Barbara Rexilius, Director *Chair's #: (518) 891-2915 Ext 302*	20 Winona Ave Box 89 Saranac Lake	12983				CC	PBL			Publication withheld			

Explanation of footnotes on page x

School Code	Name of School, Director of Program, and Phone Number	Street Address / City or Town and Zip Code	Footnotes	Type of Program	NLNAC Accreditation as of January 31, 1998	Administrative Control	Financial Support (principal source)	Number of Months in Program	Educational Requirements for Entering Adult Program	Enrollments as of October 15, 1997	Admissions Aug. 1, 1996 - July 31, 1997	Graduations Aug. 1, 1996 - July 31, 1997	Fall Admissions Aug. 1, 1997 - Dec. 31, 1997
	NEW YORK												
	- Continued												
716	Oneida BOCES PN Prog Ms Bonnie Servage, Coord *Chair's #: (315) 793-8666*	Mid Settlement Rd-Box 70 New Hartford 13413		HS		SEC SEC	PBL PBL	 22	 10	0 17	0 34	0 22	0 17
765	Onondaga & Madison BOCES Mrs Allene Rossler, Coord *Chair's #: (315) 453-4405*	4500 Crown Rd Liverpool 13090				TCH	PBL			176	136	125	136
727	Orange Ulster BOCES Mr David Barker, Supv *Chair's #: (914) 294-5431 Ext 231*	Gibson Rd Goshen 10924		HS		TCH TCH	PBL PBL	10	12 12	36 17	50 28	27 7	40 17
722	Orleans & Niagara BOCES Mrs Janet Taylor Cook, Head *Chair's #: (716) 731-4176 Ext 446*	3181 Saunders Settlement Sanborn 14132		HS		TCH TCH	PBL PBL	 20	 11	6 28	10 28	12 24	0 0
046	Oswego BOCES Sch of PN HOC Ms Carol A Ruby, Director *Chair's #: (315) 963-4263*	County Rt 64 Mexico 13114				SEC	PBL	10		54	62	49	31
725	Otsego Area Sch-Adult & Secondary Sharyn Gibbons, Head Instructor *Chair's #: (607) 286-7715*	PO Box 57 Milford 13807				SEC	PBL	10	12	24	15	30	26
739	Putnam-Westchester BOCES Mr Kevin Hart, Director *Chair's #: (914) 248-2450*	200 Boces Dr Yorktown Hts 10598				TCH	PBL	18	12	53	53	37	24
717	Rennselaer-Columbia BOCES C Bergere & S Abelson, Admins *Chair's #: (518) 273-2264*	97 Industrial Pk Rd Troy 12180				TCH	PBL			Publication withheld			
059	Rockland BOCES Mr William Renella, Principal *Chair's #: (914) 627-4770*	65 Parrot Rd West Nyack 10994		HS		TCH TCH	PBL PBL	10 20		59 1	38 0	27 2	55 6
001	Samaritan Hosp Sch of Nursing Ms Barbara Wood, Director *Chair's #: (518) 271-3285*	Burdett Ave Troy 12180				HSP	PVT			Publication withheld			
747	Schuyler-Chemung Tioga BOCES Prog Mr Stan Swider, Supv *Chair's #: (607) 739-3581 Ext 528*	459 Philo Rd Elmira 14903				TCH	PBL			60	60	50	0
726	Southern-Westchester Prog of PN Mrs Barbara Biles, Coord *Chair's #: (914) 381-0853*	310 E Boston Post Rd Mamaroneck 10543				TCH	PBL			103	103	95	104
024	St Francis PN Program Mrs Faye Weir, Dir *Chair's #: (716) 375-7315*	2221 W State St Olean 14760			A	HSP	PVT	10	12	6	12	8	10

School Code	Name of School, Director of Program, and Phone Number	Street Address / City or Town and Zip Code		Footnotes	Type of Program	NLNAC Accreditation as of January 31, 1998	Administrative Control	Financial Support (principal source)	Number of Months in Program	Educational Requirements for Entering Adult Program	Enrollments as of October 15, 1997	Admissions Aug. 1, 1996 - July 31, 1997	Graduations Aug. 1, 1996 - July 31, 1997	Fall Admissions Aug. 1, 1997 - Dec. 31, 1997
	NEW YORK													
	- Continued													
760	St Lawrence-Lewis BOCES Mrs Betty MacDonald, Coord Chair's #: (315) 353-2194	7231 State RTE 56 Norwood	13668		HS		TCH TCH	PBL PBL	20	12	61 37	48 33	21 6	33 20
711	Steuben Allegheny BOCES Prog Mr Nile Heerman, Dir Chair's #: (716) 786-3540	Rd #1, Babcock Hollow Rd Bath	14810				TCH	PBL	11	12	44	65	27	38
013	Sullivan Co BOCES Ms Kathleen Moran, Coord Chair's #: (914) 292-7900 Ext 53	85 Ferndale Looms Rd Liberty	12754				SEC	PBL			Publication withheld			
010	Syracuse Central Tech Voc Center Mrs Margaret O'Connor, Coord Chair's #: (315) 435-4316	258 E Adams St Syracuse	13202		HSE		TCH TCH	PBL PBL	10 30	12 12	51 26	75 18	41 1	28 14
081	Ulster BOCES Sch of PN Mrs Diane Davies, Admin Chair's #: (914) 331-6680 Ext 232	PO Box 601 Port Ewen	12466		HS		TCH TCH	PBL PBL	12	12 12	99 24	129 28	101 12	103 24
070	Voc Ed & Extn Bd-Nassau Co Sch Mrs Mary F Watson, Supervisor Chair's #: (516) 572-1704 Ext 234	899-A Jerusalem Ave Uniondale	11553			A	TCH	PVT	11	12	200	204	156	200
769	Wa-War'N-Hmltn Essex BOCES Mrs Sharon M Erbe, Coord Chair's #: (518) 746-3428	Dix Ave Hudson Falls	12839		HSE		TCH TCH	PBL PBL	11 17	12 12	22 71	29 53	25 23	22 44
023	Wayne-Finger Lakes BOCES (2 Branch Ms Beverlyann Zier, Dir Chair's #: (315) 331-2346	4440 E Ridge Rd Williamson	14589				TCH	PBL			42	81	55	60
766	Westchester Comm College Mrs Marie Cahill, Chair Chair's #: (914) 785-6884	75 Grasslands Rd Valhalla	10595				CC	PBL	11	12	29	50	41	50
055	Western Suffolk BOCES Ms Eileen Anetrella, Principal Chair's #: (516) 261-3600 Ext 202	Laurel Hill Rd Northport	11768		HSE	A A	TCH TCH	PBL PBL	10 20	12 12	129 25	123 20	79 1	78 30
	NORTH CAROLINA													
	28 Programs in 28 Schools													
047	Anson Comm College Mrs Sarah U Lee, Chair Chair's #: (704) 272-7635 Ext 252	PO Box 126 Polkton	28135				CC	PBL	12	12	17	22	12	20
011	Asheville-Buncombe Tech Comm Colle Mrs Brenda Causey, Interim Chair Chair's #: (704) 254-1921 Ext 262	340 Victoria Rd Asheville	28801				TCH	PBL	12	12	39	45	38	42

School Code	Name of School, Director of Program, and Phone Number	Street Address, City or Town and Zip Code		Footnotes	Type of Program	NLNAC Accreditation as of January 31, 1998	Administrative Control	Financial Support (principal source)	Number of Months in Program	Educational Requirements for Entering Adult Program	Enrollments as of October 15, 1997	Admissions Aug. 1, 1996 - July 31, 1997	Graduations Aug. 1, 1996 - July 31, 1997	Fall Admissions Aug. 1, 1997 - Dec. 31, 1997
	NORTH CAROLINA													
	- Continued													
014	Beaufort Co Comm College Ms Carolyn Lee, Director *Chair's #: (919) 946-6194 Ext 318*	PO Box 1069 Washington	27889				CC	PBL	12	12	20	20	15	20
901	Bladen Comm College Mrs Saundra Meares, Chair *Chair's #: (910) 862-2164 Ext 316*	PO Box 266 Dublin	28332				CC	PBL	12	12	16	16	15	16
067	Brunswick Comm College Ms Connie Milliken, Director *Chair's #: (910) 754-6900 Ext 350*	PO Box 30 Supply	28462				CC	PBL	12	12	23	22	21	23
032	Cape Fear Comm College Ms Vinson Greene, Director *Chair's #: (910) 251-5190 Ext 8482*	411 N Front St Wilmington	28401				CC	PBL			Publication withheld			
035	Carteret Comm College Mrs Nancy McBride, Coord *Chair's #: (919) 247-6000 Ext 170*	3505 Arendell St Morehead City	28557				CC	PBL	12	12	22	20	16	24
069	Central Carolina Comm College Mrs Rhonda Evans, Chair *Chair's #: (919) 775-5401 Ext 281*	Route 1 Box 447-C Lillington	27546	7			CC	PBL	12	12	35	37	24	35
015	Cleveland Comm College Ms Katherine Jones, Dept Head *Chair's #: (704) 484-4001*	137 S Post Rd Shelby	28150				CC	PBL			28	22	16	20
036	Coastal Carolina Comm College Mrs Paula V Gribble, Chair *Chair's #: (910) 938-6269*	444 Western Blvd Jacksonville	28540				CC	PBL	12	12	18	20	17	0
013	Coll of the Albemarle Mrs Elizabeth Jones, Coord *Chair's #: (919) 335-0821 Ext 289*	PO Box 2327 Elizabeth City	27906				CC	PBL	12	12	19	18	13	19
033	Craven Comm College Mrs Carolyn Jones, Director *Chair's #: (919) 638-7342*	800 College Court New Bern	28562				CC	PBL	12		20	20	16	20
004	Durham Tech Comm College Dr Louise J Gooche, Director *Chair's #: (919) 686-3673*	1637 Lawson St Durham	27703				TCH	PBL	12	12	40	40	30	20
023	Fayetteville Tech Comm College Mrs Kathy T Weeks, Chair *Chair's #: (910) 678-8482*	PO Box 35236 Fayetteville	28303				CC	PBL	11	12	28	21	24	24
012	Forsyth Tech Comm College Mrs Carolyn Rajacich, Asst Dean *Chair's #: (910) 723-0371 Ext 7416*	2100 Silas Creek Pkwy Winston-Salem	27103				CC	PBL			Publication withheld			

School Code	Name of School, Director of Program, and Phone Number	Street Address, City or Town and Zip Code		Footnotes	Type of Program	NLNAC Accreditation as of January 31, 1998	Administrative Control	Financial Support (principal source)	Number of Months in Program	Educational Requirements for Entering Adult Program	Enrollments as of October 15, 1997	Admissions Aug. 1, 1996 - July 31, 1997	Graduations Aug. 1, 1996 - July 31, 1997	Fall Admissions Aug. 1, 1997 - Dec. 31, 1997
	NORTH CAROLINA													
	- Continued													
060	Gaston College Mrs Beverly Davis, Chair *Chair's #: (704) 922-6400*	1 Timken Dr Lincolnton	28092				CC	PBL	12	12	32	30	19	32
055	Isothermal Comm College Ms Debbie Sain Rogers, Director *Chair's #: (704) 286-3636 Ext 254*	PO Box 804 Spindale	28160	7			CC	PBL	12	12	24	24	23	24
005	James Sprunt Comm Coll Mrs Rhonda B Ferrell, Chair *Chair's #: (910) 296-2450*	PO Box 398 Kenansville	28349				CC	PBL	12	12	19	20	14	20
056	Lenoir Comm College Mrs Alexis Welch, Dean *Chair's #: (919) 527-6223 Ext 801*	PO Box 188 Kinston	28502				CC	PBL	12	12	17	19	10	14
062	McDowell Tech Comm Coll Mrs Christine Tugwell, Dir *Chair's #: (704) 652-6021 Ext 711*	Rt #1, Box 170 Marion	28752				CC	PBL	12	12	20	20	16	20
049	Montgomery Comm College Mrs Deborah B Morton, Director *Chair's #: (910) 576-6222 Ext 205*	PO Box 787 Troy	27371				TCH	PBL	12	12	30	28	20	25
070	Rockingham Comm College Mrs Cathy Franklin-Griffin, Dean *Chair's #: (910) 342-4261 Ext 248*	PO Box 38 Wentworth	27375				CC	PBL		Publication withheld				
042	Sampson Comm Coll Mrs Mary Brown, Chair *Chair's #: (910) 592-8081 Ext 439*	PO Drawer 318 Clinton	28328				CC	PBL	12	12	20	20	20	20
058	Sandhills Comm College-Nsg Dept Ms Star Mitchell, Chair *Chair's #: (910) 692-6185 Ext 606*	2200 Airport Rd Pinehurst	28374				CC	PBL		Publication withheld				
043	Southeastern Comm College Mrs Peggy Blackmon, Dean *Chair's #: (910) 642-7141 Ext 240*	PO Box 151 Whiteville	28472				CC	PBL	12	12	24	25	7	25
006	Surry Comm Coll Ms Sharon S Kallam, Chair *Chair's #: (910) 386-8121 Ext 227*	PO Box 304 Dobson	27017				CC	PBL	12	12	23	30	20	30
052	Vance-Granville Comm College Mrs Jo Anne Alston, Chair *Chair's #: (919) 492-2061 Ext 307*	PO Box 917 Henderson	27536	7			TCH	PBL		Data reported w/AD prog				
007	Wayne Comm College Dr Cynthia B Archie, Head *Chair's #: (919) 735-5151 Ext 297*	Box 8002 Goldsboro	27533				CC	PBL	12	12	18	19	7	18

Explanation of footnotes on page x

School Code	Name of School, Director of Program, and Phone Number	Street Address / City or Town and Zip Code		Footnotes	Type of Program	NLNAC Accreditation as of January 31, 1998	Administrative Control	Financial Support (principal source)	Number of Months in Program	Educational Requirements for Entering Adult Program	Enrollments as of October 15, 1997	Admissions Aug. 1, 1996 - July 31, 1997	Graduations Aug. 1, 1996 - July 31, 1997	Fall Admissions Aug. 1, 1997 - Dec. 31, 1997
	NORTH DAKOTA													
	6 Programs in 6 Schools													
007	Dickinson State Univ Dr Sandra Affeldt, Chair *Chair's #: (701) 227-2172*	291 Campus Dr Dickinson	58601	7		A	CC	PBL			Data reported w/AD prog			
005	Fort Berthold Comm Coll Mrs Brenda Caranicas, Director *Chair's #: (701) 627-4738 Ext 254*	PO Box 490 New Town	58763	7			CC	PBL	18	12	24	16	10	12
004	North Dakota State College of Science Mrs Marlys Baumann, Chair *Chair's #: (701) 671-2967 Ext 2968*	800 6th N Wahpeton	58075			A	CC	PBL	18	12	109	45	42	27
900	Northwest Technical Coll Ms Mary Wiersma, Director *Chair's #: (218) 773-4556*	Highway 220 W East Grand Forks	56721				TCH	PBL			Also reports in MN			
009	United Tribes Tech College Dr Kathryn Zimmer, Director *Chair's #: (701) 255-3285 Ext 265*	3315 University Dr Bismarck	58504			A	CC	PVT	17	12	62	35	13	35
012	Univ of North Dakota-Williston Ms Linda Tharp, Chair *Chair's #: (701) 774-4290*	1410 Univ Ave Box 1326 Williston	58802				CC	PBL			22	24	18	0
	OHIO													
	43 Programs in 40 Schools													
001	Akron Sch of Practical Nursing Mrs Marilyn Barkley, Dir *Chair's #: (330) 761-3255*	619 Sumner St Akron	44311			A	SEC	PBL	11	12	60	60	54	60
015	Apollo Sch of PN Miss Ruth Speakman, Coord *Chair's #: (419) 998-2975*	3325 Shawnee Rd Lima	45806				TCH	PBL	10		33	39	30	34
026	Belmont Tech College-Sch of PN Mrs Rebecca Kurtz, Asst Dean *Chair's #: (614) 695-9500 Ext 24*	120 Fox-Shannon Pl St Clairsville	43950				TCH	PBL	12	12	25	35	32	22
021	Butler Co Program of PN Ed Mrs Joyce Harris, Dir *Chair's #: (513) 868-6300 Ext 4203*	3603 Hamilton-Middletown Hamilton	45011				TCH	PBL	10		98	106	79	68
004	Central Sch of Practical Nursing, Inc Ms Nancy Giesser, Dir *Chair's #: (216) 391-8434*	4600 Carnegie Ave Cleveland	44103			A	IND	PVT	12	12	63	84	55	42
010	Choffin Sch of Practical Nursing Mrs Janet M Carpenter, Supv *Chair's #: (330) 744-8722*	200 East Wood St Youngstown	44503			A	TCH	PBL	10	12	55	58	52	57

School Code	Name of School, Director of Program, and Phone Number	Street Address / City or Town and Zip Code		Footnotes	Type of Program	NLNAC Accreditation as of January 31, 1998	Administrative Control	Financial Support (principal source)	Number of Months in Program	Educational Requirements for Entering Adult Program	Enrollments as of October 15, 1997	Admissions Aug. 1, 1996 - July 31, 1997	Graduations Aug. 1, 1996 - July 31, 1997	Fall Admissions Aug. 1, 1997 - Dec. 31, 1997
	OHIO													
	- Continued													
002	Cincinnati Public Sch of PN Ms Roberta Russo, Director *Chair's #: (513) 977-8082*	425 Ezzard Charles Dr Cincinnati	45203				TCH	PBL	11	12	55	90	50	31
033	Clark State Comm College Mrs Carolyn Swanger, Dean *Chair's #: (937) 328-6060*	570 E Leffel Ln Box 570 Springfield	45501				TCH	PBL	11	12	30	36	22	35
058	Collins Career Center Mrs Lola Cress, Dir *Chair's #: (614) 532-7187*	11627 St RT 243 Chesapeake	45619				TCH	PBL	11	12	32	36	24	36
012	Columbus Pub Schools - Sch of PN Ms Jill Whalen, Coord *Chair's #: (614) 365-5241*	100 Arcadia Ave Rm-300 W Columbus	43202				SEC	PBL			72	78	57	30
009	Cuyahoga Comm College--PN Prog Mrs Janice Melnick, Interim Manager *Chair's #: (216) 987-2276*	4250 Richmond Rd Cleveland	44122	7			CC	PBL			Data reported w/AD prog			
019	EHOVE Sch of PN Ms Deborah Toth, Dir *Chair's #: (419) 627-9665 Ext 284*	316 West Mason Rd Milan	44846	2			TCH	PBL			34	34	29	33
014	Great Oaks Sch of PN Scarlet Oaks Care Mrs Lina Nichols, Dir *Chair's #: (513) 771-8810 Ext 429*	3254 E Kemper Rd Cincinnati	45241			A	TCH	PBL	11	12	99	95	61	67
017	Hannah E Mullins Sch of Practical Nsg Mrs Beverly Henderson, Coord *Chair's #: (330) 332-8940*	1200 E 6 th Salem	44460			A	SEC	PBL			Publication withheld			
040	Hocking Tech College Nsg Career Ladd Mrs Nadine Goebel, Dean *Chair's #: (614) 753-3591 Ext 2215*	3301 Hocking Pkwy Nelsonville	45764			A	TCH	PBL	12	12	223	228	160	66
047	Jefferson Comm Coll Miss Kathleen F Keenan, Director *Chair's #: (614) 264-5591*	4000 Sunset Blvd Steubenville	43952				TCH	PBL			Publication withheld			
055	Knoedler Sch of PN Ed Mrs Dawn Bleau, Dir *Chair's #: (440) 576-6015 Ext 201*	1565 Rt 167 Jefferson	44047				TCH	PBL	11	12	44	39	32	45
053	Knox Co Career Center Mrs Waynette Bridwell, Coord *Chair's #: (614) 397-5820 Ext 269*	306 Martinsburg Rd Mt Vernon	43050				TCH	PBL	12	12	33	29	24	32
041	Lorain County Comm College PN Progr Mr Robert A Schloss, Dir *Chair's #: (440) 366-4016 Ext 4016*	1005 N Abbe Rd Elyria	44035			A	CC	PBL	11	12	61	62	48	0

Explanation of footnotes on page x

School Code	Name of School, Director of Program, and Phone Number	Street Address / City or Town and Zip Code	Footnotes	Type of Program	NLNAC Accreditation as of January 31, 1998	Administrative Control	Financial Support (principal source)	Number of Months in Program	Educational Requirements for Entering Adult Program	Enrollments as of October 15, 1997	Admissions Aug. 1, 1996 - July 31, 1997	Graduations Aug. 1, 1996 - July 31, 1997	Fall Admissions Aug. 1, 1997 - Dec. 31, 1997
	OHIO												
	- Continued												
006	Marymount Sch of Practical Nursing Ms Susan Leonard, Dir Chair's #: (216) 587-8160 Ext 2439	12300 McCracken Rd Garfield Hts 44125			A	HSP	PVT	12	12	27	31	27	36
003	Miami Valley Career Tech Ms Frances Childers, Dir Chair's #: (513) 854-6370	6800 Hoke Rd Clayton 45315				TCH	PBL			Publication withheld			
039	Mid-East OH Voc Sch Syst Adult&Cont Mrs Cathy Learn, Coord Chair's #: (740) 455-3111 Ext 147	400 Richards Rd Zanesville 43701	HS			TCH TCH	PBL PBL	11 21	12 12	49 31	43 18	36 13	50 19
044	Muskingum Perry Career Center Mrs Cathy Learn, Coord Chair's #: (740) 455-3111 Ext 147	400 Richards Rd Zanesville 43701	HS			TCH TCH	PBL PBL	11 21	12 12	49 31	43 18	36 13	50 19
052	North Central Tech College Ms Carol Lepley, Director Chair's #: (419) 755-4823	2441 Kenwood Circle Box 698 Mansfield 44901				CC	PBL	12	12	53	66	51	28
048	Northwest St Comm College Mrs Karen Short, Coord Chair's #: (419) 267-5511 Ext 253	22 600 St Rt 34 Archbold 43502				CC	PBL	12	12	36	47	33	38
061	Ohio Hi-Point Joint Voc Sch of PN Ms Darlene C Chiles, Supv Chair's #: (937) 599-6275 Ext 210	2280 State Rt 540 Bellefontaine 43311				TCH	PBL	12	12	36	36	21	36
030	Parma Sch of PN Mrs Myrna George, Supv Chair's #: (440) 885-2364	6726 Ridge Rd Parma 44129				TCH	PBL			Publication withheld			
065	Pickaway-Ross Co JVSD Mrs Mary Van Sickle, Coord Chair's #: (614) 773-6873	Bldg 4 17273 St Rd 104 Chillicothe 45601			A	TCH	PBL	10	12	31	39	34	36
037	PN Program of Canton City Schs Mrs Judy Stauder, Coord Chair's #: (330) 453-3271	1253 Third St SE Canton 44707			A	SEC	PBL	12	12	50	71	48	63
051	PN Program of Scioto Co JVS Ms Brenda J Horr, Director Chair's #: (614) 259-5522	PO Box 766 Lucasville 45648				TCH	PBL			Publication withheld			
050	PN Sch-Buckeye Hills Career Ctr Mrs Phyllis Pope-Brown, Coord Chair's #: (614) 245-5334 Ext 206	PO Box 157 351 Buckeye Hills Rio Grande 45674				TCH	PBL	12	12	45	45	27	0
034	Portage Lakes Car Ctr W Howard Nicol Mrs Mary Ann Cosgarea, Coord Chair's #: (330) 896-8105	4401 Shriver Rd PO Box 248 Green 44232				TCH	PBL	11	12	34	32	27	34

Explanation of footnotes on page x

School Code	Name of School, Director of Program, and Phone Number	Street Address / City or Town and Zip Code		Footnotes	Type of Program	NLNAC Accreditation as of January 31, 1998	Administrative Control	Financial Support (principal source)	Number of Months in Program	Educational Requirements for Entering Adult Program	Enrollments as of October 15, 1997	Admissions Aug. 1, 1996 - July 31, 1997	Graduations Aug. 1, 1996 - July 31, 1997	Fall Admissions Aug. 1, 1997 - Dec. 31, 1997
	OHIO													
	- Continued													
060	Southern State Comm College Mrs Jo Carol Laymon, Director *Chair's #: (937) 393-3431 Ext 2640*	200 Hobart Dr Hillsboro	45133				CC	PBL	11	12	26	39	22	0
020	The Stautzenberger Coll Ms Jane Ridge, Coord *Chair's #: (419) 423-2211*	1637 Tiffine Ave Findlay	45840	2			IND	PVT			85	0	59	57
008	Toledo Sch of PN-Woodward Ms Veronica Backman, Coord *Chair's #: (419) 244-8301*	1602 Washington St Toledo	43624				SEC	PBL			Publication withheld			
016	Tri-Rivers Sch of PN Dr Judith R Higel, Manager *Chair's #: (614) 389-6347*	2222 Marion Mt Gilead Rd Marion	43302				TCH	PBL	10	12	45	59	52	55
067	Trumbull Co Joint Voc Sch Mrs Linda Reader, Coord *Chair's #: (330) 847-0503 Ext 327*	528 Education Highway Warren	44483		HS		TCH TCH	PBL PBL	18	12	12 25	4 13	1 8	7 17
054	Upper Valley Joint Voc Sch of PN Ms Doris Luckett, Director *Chair's #: (937) 778-1980 Ext 253*	8811 Career Dr Piqua	45356				TCH	PBL	12	12	42	77	31	20
023	Washington State Comm College Mrs Ann Stewart, Administrator *Chair's #: (740) 374-8716 Ext 671*	710 Colegate Dr Marietta	45750				CC	PBL			36	36	30	36
046	Wayne Adult Sch of PN (2 Progs) Mrs Kathy Sommers, Coord *Chair's #: (330) 669-2134 Ext 209*	518 W Prospect St Smithville	44677		HS		SEC SEC	PBL PBL	12 18	12 12	52 0	38 16	28 12	38 25
036	Willoughby-Eastlk Sch of PN (2 Progs) Mrs Barbara Sesler, Dir *Chair's #: (440) 946-7085 Ext 1*	25 Public Square Willoughby	44094		HS		SEC SEC	PBL PBL	11 18	12 12	26 22	24 20	24 11	26 22
	OKLAHOMA													
	31 Programs in 31 Schools													
022	Autry Technology Center Mrs Barbara Simmons, Coord *Chair's #: (405) 242-2750 Ext 163*	1201 W Willow Enid	73073			A	TCH	PBL	12	12	20	20	15	0
035	Caddo-Kiowa Area Voc-Tech Sch Dist 2 Ms Marquita Lindsey, Coord *Chair's #: (405) 643-5511 Ext 263*	PO Box 90 Ft Cobb	73015			A	TCH	PBL	14	12	35	30	20	16
027	Canadian Valley Area AVTS-Dist 6 Mrs Lois A Robinson, Coord *Chair's #: (405) 422-2217*	6505 E Hwy 66 El Reno	73036			A	TCH	PBL	12	12	19	24	21	24

Explanation of footnotes on page x

School Code	Name of School, Director of Program, and Phone Number	Street Address City or Town and Zip Code		Footnotes	Type of Program	NLNAC Accreditation as of January 31, 1998	Administrative Control	Financial Support (principal source)	Number of Months in Program	Educational Requirements for Entering Adult Program	Enrollments as of October 15, 1997	Admissions Aug. 1, 1996 - July 31, 1997	Graduations Aug. 1, 1996 - July 31, 1997	Fall Admissions Aug. 1, 1997 - Dec. 31, 1997
	OKLAHOMA													
	- Continued													
021	Canadian Valley AVTS Ms Bernadette Burns, Director *Chair's #: (405) 224-7220 Ext 592*	1401 Michigan Ave Chichasha	73018			A	TCH	PBL			Publication withheld			
024	Central OK Area Voc-Tech Sch Dist 3 Ms Carla J Brittenham, Coord *Chair's #: (918) 352-2551 Ext 288*	3 C T Circle Drumright	74030			A	TCH	PBL	12	12	46	49	34	24
076	Chisholm Trail Area Voc-Tech Sch Mrs Carla Maloy, Coord *Chair's #: (405) 729-8324*	Rt 1 Box 60 Omega	73764			A	TCH	PBL	11	12	13	12	9	14
063	Demarge College Mrs Sandi White, Dir *Chair's #: (405) 692-6409 Ext 23*	3608 H W 58th St Oklahoma City	73142	1		IND	PVT		12	11	45	50	33	45
042	Francis Tuttle Voc-Tech Ctr PN Prog Mrs Linda Dawkins, Coord *Chair's #: (405) 717-4128*	12777 N Rockwell Oklahoma City	73142			A	TCH	PBL	11	12	31	31	30	24
026	Gordon Cooper Technology Center Mrs Lisa Morlan, Coord *Chair's #: (405) 273-7493 Ext 291*	One John C Bruton Blvd Shawnee	74801				TCH	PBL	11	12	26	26	18	26
010	GPAVTS Dist 9 Ms LaDonna Meyer, Dir *Chair's #: (580) 250-5595*	4500 W Lee Blvd Lawton	73505			A	TCH	PBL	12	12	30	60	50	30
900	Green Country AVTS Ms Molly Parker, Director *Chair's #: (918) 758-0840*	PO Box 1217 Okmulgee	74047				TCH	PBL	12	12	18	20	17	0
012	High Plains AVTS Sch of PN Ms Sue Mitchell, Dir *Chair's #: (405) 571-6159*	3921 34th St Woodward	73801				TCH	PBL			Publication withheld			
011	Indian Captl Voc-Tech Sch (3 Campuses) Mrs Debra A Bartel, Coord *Chair's #: (918) 775-9119 Ext 108*	H C 61 Box 12 Sallisaw	74955			A	TCH	PBL	15	12	78	78	61	0
039	Kiamichi Area Voc-Tech (6 Campuses) Mrs Sherry Payne Burke, Director *Chair's #: (918) 567-2264*	Rt 2 Box 1800 Talihina	74571			A	TCH	PBL	12	12	142	144	140	144
032	Meridian Technology Center Mrs Dolores Cotton, Coord *Chair's #: (405) 377-3333 Ext 324*	1312 S Sangre Rd Stillwater	74074			A	TCH	PBL	12	12	36	29	27	26
004	Metro Area Voc Technical School Mrs Nettie Seale, Coord *Chair's #: (405) 424-8324 Ext 610*	1720 Springlake Dr Oklahoma City	73111			A	TCH	PBL	12	12	42	22	42	42

Explanation of footnotes on page x

OKLAHOMA

- Continued

School Code	Name of School, Director of Program, and Phone Number	Street Address / City or Town and Zip Code	Footnotes	Type of Program	NLNAC Accreditation as of January 31, 1998	Administrative Control	Financial Support (principal source)	Number of Months in Program	Educational Requirements for Entering Adult Program	Enrollments as of October 15, 1997	Admissions Aug. 1, 1996 - July 31, 1997	Graduations Aug. 1, 1996 - July 31, 1997	Fall Admissions Aug. 1, 1997 - Dec. 31, 1997
030	Mid-America Area Voc-Tech Sch Dist 8 Mrs Gina Doyle, Coord *Chair's #: (405) 449-3391 Ext 265*	PO Box H Wayne 73095			A	TCH	PBL	11	12	27	28	24	28
017	Mid-Del Lewis Eubanks AVTS Mrs Vivian Bingman, Dir *Chair's #: (405) 739-1713 Ext 314*	1621 Maple Dr Midwest City 73110	 HSE		A A	TCH TCH	PBL PBL	0 16	12 12	30 21	17 10	13 6	16 23
020	Moore-Norman Area V-T Sch Dist 17 Ms Naomi R Jones, Director *Chair's #: (405) 364-5763 Ext 349*	4701 12th Ave NW Norman 73069			A	TCH	PBL	10	12	46	55	48	48
029	Northeast Area Voc-Tech Sch (3 Campu Ms Teresa Fraizer, Coord *Chair's #: (918) 825-5555*	PO Box 487 Pryor 74362			A	TCH	PBL	11	12	57	69	56	66
031	Pioneer Area Voc-Tech Sch Dist 13 Mrs Mary E Frantz, Coord *Chair's #: (580) 762-8336 Ext 251*	2101 N Ash Ponca City 74601				TCH	PBL	11	12	27	25	21	27
001	Platt College Ms Kay Haywood, Dir *Chair's #: (405) 946-7799 Ext 23*	309 S Ann Arbor Ave Oklahoma City 73128	1			TCH	PVT			Publication withheld			
008	Pontotoc County Skills Center Mrs Penny Stone, Dir *Chair's #: (405) 436-0180 Ext 2258*	601 W 33rd Ada 74820				TCH	PBL			Publication withheld			
033	Red River Area V-T Sch Dist 19 Mrs Earlene K Werner, Dir *Chair's #: (580) 255-2903 Ext 237*	PO Box 1807 Duncan 73533			A	TCH	PBL	12	12	25	26	17	26
023	School of Tech Training Mr Paul Deweese, Dir *Chair's #: (405) 355-4416*	112 S W 11th St Lawton 73501	1			TCH	PVT	12	12	38	30	15	16
019	Southern Oklahoma Area Voc-Tech Ctr Ms Sylvia Diggs, Coord *Chair's #: (580) 223-2070*	Rt 1 Box 14M Ardmore 73401				TCH	PBL			Publication withheld			
043	Southwest OK Sch PN Mrs Elva Pruitt, Dir *Chair's #: (405) 477-2250 Ext 257*	1121 North Spurgeon Altus 73521				TCH	PBL	12	12	23	28	23	0
005	Tri-Co Area Voc-Tech Sch Dist 1 Mrs Ruth Howell, Dir *Chair's #: (918) 331-3223*	6101 Nowata Rd Bartlesville 74006			A	TCH	PBL	11	12	24	27	33	0
009	Tulsa Technology Center Ms Rita Hejtmanick, Coord *Chair's #: (918) 828-1043*	3420 S Memorial Dr Tulsa 74145			A	TCH	PBL	12	12	32	35	31	35

Explanation of footnotes on page x

School Code	Name of School, Director of Program, and Phone Number	Street Address, City or Town and Zip Code	Footnotes	Type of Program	NLNAC Accreditation as of January 31, 1998	Administrative Control	Financial Support (principal source)	Number of Months in Program	Educational Requirements for Entering Adult Program	Enrollments as of October 15, 1997	Admissions Aug. 1, 1996 - July 31, 1997	Graduations Aug. 1, 1996 - July 31, 1997	Fall Admissions Aug. 1, 1997 - Dec. 31, 1997
	OKLAHOMA												
	- Continued												
045	Wes Watkins Area Voc Tech Mrs Roberta Jeffrey, Coord *Chair's #: (405) 452-5500 Ext 277*	Route 2 Box 159-1 Wetumka 74883				TCH	PBL	12	12	20	26	15	2
028	Western Technology Center Mrs Marianne Doss, Coord *Chair's #: (580) 562-3181 Ext 2264*	PO Box 1469 621 Sooner Dr Burns Flat 73624			A	TCH	PBL	12	12	34	36	31	36
	OREGON												
	11 Programs in 11 Schools												
009	Blue Mountain Comm College PN Prog Mrs Elizabeth Sullivan, Chair *Chair's #: (541) 278-5379*	PO Box 100 Pendleton 97801	7			CC	PBL			Data reported w/AD prog			
004	Central Oregon Comm College PN Prog Mr Doug McCready, Dir *Chair's #: (541) 383-7546*	2600 NW College Way Bend 97701	7			CC	PBL			Data reported w/AD prog			
007	Chemeketa Comm College Dr Doris Williams, Dir *Chair's #: (503) 399-5058*	4000 Lancaster Dr, NE Salem 97309	7			CC	PBL			Data repoorted w/AD prog			
016	Clackamas Comm College PN Prog Mrs Arlene Jurgens, Chair *Chair's #: (503) 657-6958 Ext 2428*	19600 S Molalla Ave Oregon City 97045	7			CC	PBL			Data reported w/AD prog			
017	Clatsop Comm College Ms Karen M Burke, Dir *Chair's #: (503) 338-2496*	16th & Jerome Astoria 97103	7			CC	PBL			Data reported w/AD prog			
006	Lane Comm College PN Prog Ms Joyce Godels, Chair *Chair's #: (503) 747-4501 Ext 2619*	4000 E 30th Ave Eugene 97405	7			CC	PBL			Data reported w/AD Prog			
015	Mt Hood Comm College PN Prog Dr Joan Carley Oliver, Dir *Chair's #: (503) 667-7404*	26000 SE Stark Gresham 97030	7			CC	PBL			Data reported w/AD prog			
010	Rogue Comm College Mrs Linda Wagner, Director *Chair's #: (541) 471-3500 Ext 268*	3345 Redwood Hwy Grants Pass 97527	7			CC	PBL			Data reported w/AD prog			
013	Treasure Valley Comm College PN Prog Mrs Maureen McDonough, Director *Chair's #: (541) 889-6493 Ext 345*	650 College Blvd Ontario 97914	7			CC	PBL			Data reported w/AD Prog			
014	Umpqua Comm College PN Prog Mr Duane D Alexenko, Dir *Chair's #: (541) 440-4613*	PO Box 967 Roseburg 97470	7			CC	PBL			Data reported w/AD prog			

PENNSYLVANIA

49 Programs in 49 Schools

School Code	Name of School, Director of Program, and Phone Number	Street Address / City or Town and Zip Code	Footnotes	Type of Program	NLNAC Accreditation as of January 31, 1998	Administrative Control	Financial Support (principal source)	Number of Months in Program	Educational Requirements for Entering Adult Program	Enrollments as of October 15, 1997	Admissions Aug. 1, 1996 - July 31, 1997	Graduations Aug. 1, 1996 - July 31, 1997	Fall Admissions Aug. 1, 1997 - Dec. 31, 1997
055	Career Tech Center of Lakawanna Co, Mrs Sallie Noto, Supv, Chair's #: (717) 346-8728	3201 Rockwell Ave, Scranton 18508			A	TCH	PBL	12	12	57	40	45	30
031	Alvernia School-St Francis Med Center, Miss Lois McKinley, Dir, Chair's #: (412) 622-4496	400 45th St, Pittsburgh 15201			A	HSP	PVT	12	12	13	27	15	0
021	Bucks County Technical School, Dr Patricia Duick, Coord, Chair's #: (215) 949-1700 Ext 32	610 Wistar Rd, Fairless Hills 19030			A	TCH	PBL	11	12	76	38	32	38
013	Center for Arts & Technology, Jane M Alexander, Dir, Chair's #: (610) 384-1585 Ext 216	1635 E Lincoln Hwy, Coatesville 19320			A	TCH	PBL	15	12	75	50	40	50
057	Central Susquehanna Career Center, Ms Kay Yannallone, Acting Dir, Chair's #: (717) 437-3176	DeLong Building Box 140, Washingtonville 17884			A	GOV	PBL	12		75	88	76	36
018	Centre County Area Voc Tech Sch, Mrs Ellouise Garver, Coord, Chair's #: (814) 359-2582 Ext 265	540 N Harrison Rd, Pleasant Gap 16823			A	TCH	PBL	12	12	16	26	22	21
009	Chester-Upland Sch Dist, Ms Lucy E Yates, Coord, Chair's #: (610) 447-3830	200 West 9th St Rm A109, Chester 19013	2			SEC	PBL			Publication withheld			
074	Clarion Co Area Voc-Tech School, Mrs Barbara Barger, Coord, Chair's #: (814) 226-5857	1976 Career Way, Shippenville 16254			A	TCH	PBL	12	12	24	30	28	36
068	Clearfield Co Area Voc Tech School, Mrs Barbara A Tubbs, Supervisor, Chair's #: (814) 765-4047 Ext 1111	RR #1 Box 5, Clearfield 16830			A	TCH	PBL	12	12	33	38	28	18
051	Comm College of Beaver County, Mrs Linda Gallagher, Dir, Chair's #: (412) 775-8561 Ext 200	1 Campus Dr, Monaca 15061	7			CC	PBL			Data reported w/AD Prog			
064	Crawford County Area Voc Tech School, Dr Carol Vogt, Dir, Chair's #: (814) 724-6028	860 Thurston Rd, Meadville 16335			A	TCH	PBL	12	12	17	15	29	21
002	Delaware Co Area Voc-Tech Sch, Mrs Catherine Coakley, Coord, Chair's #: (610) 583-2934 Ext 221	Delmar Dr & Henderson Blvd, Folcroft 19032			A	TCH	PBL	12	12	52	32	32	36
044	Eastern Center for Arts and Technology, Mrs Barbara Gravel, Supervisor, Chair's #: (215) 784-4805	3075 Terwood Rd, Willow Grove 19090			A	TCH	PBL	12	12	52	19	56	21

Explanation of footnotes on page x

PENNSYLVANIA
- Continued

School Code	Name of School, Director of Program, and Phone Number	Street Address / City or Town and Zip Code	Footnotes	Type of Program	NLNAC Accreditation as of January 31, 1998	Administrative Control	Financial Support (principal source)	Number of Months in Program	Educational Requirements for Entering Adult Program	Enrollments as of October 15, 1997	Admissions Aug. 1, 1996 - July 31, 1997	Graduations Aug. 1, 1996 - July 31, 1997	Fall Admissions Aug. 1, 1997 - Dec. 31, 1997
043	Fayette Co Area Voc Tech School Mrs Marilyn Tyhonas, Coord *Chair's #: (412) 437-2724 Ext 23*	RD #2, Box 122A Uniontown 15401			A	TCH	PBL	12	12	48	58	50	19
900	Forbes Rd East Area Voc Tech School Mrs Edna Litwiller, Coord *Chair's #: (412) 373-8100 Ext 232*	607 Beatty Rd Monroeville 15146				TCH	PBL	12	12	26	23	18	0
019	Franklin Co Career and Tech Center Mrs Mary E Butts, Admin *Chair's #: (717) 263-5667*	2463 Loop Rd Chambersburg 17201			A	TCH	PBL	12	12	72	78	70	38
032	Greater Altoona Career Tech Center Mrs Margaret O'Brien, Coord *Chair's #: (814) 946-8490*	1500 4th Ave Altoona 16602				TCH	PBL	12	12	34	42	30	37
005	Greater Johnstown Area Voc Tech Scho Mrs Bonnie Ford, Coord *Chair's #: (814) 269-4393*	445 Schoolhouse Rd Johnstown 15904			A	TCH	PVT	12	12	51	42	38	39
067	Greene County Area Voc Tech School Mrs Patsy Trump, Coord *Chair's #: (412) 627-3106 Ext 207*	60 Zimmerman Dr Waynesburg 15370			A	TCH	PBL	12	12	28	32	12	14
041	Hanover Public School Dist Mrs Shirley LeDane, Coord *Chair's #: (717) 637-2111 Ext 204*	403 Moul Ave Hanover 17331			A	SEC	PVT	12	12	45	40	40	0
084	Harrisburg Area Comm College Mr Ronald Rebuck, Coord *Chair's #: (717) 780-2344*	One HACC Dr Harrisburg 17110			A	CC	PBL	12	12	32	40	34	40
066	Hazleton Area Voc Tech School Ms Bernice Platek, Coord *Chair's #: (717) 459-3172*	1451 West 23rd St Hazleton 18201			A	TCH	PVT	12	12	28	23	23	28
062	Indiana Co Area Voc-Tech School Mrs Sharon Powell Laney, Coord *Chair's #: (412) 349-6700 Ext 121*	441 Hamill Rd Indiana 15701			A	TCH	PBL			Publication withheld			
053	Jefferson Co-Dubois Area Voc Tech Sch Mrs Marion Monahan, Coord *Chair's #: (814) 653-8265*	100 Jeff Tech Dr Reynoldsville 15851			A	TCH	PBL	12	12	18	48	22	24
065	Juniata-Mifflin Co Area Voc Tech Sch Ms Marcia Dedmon, Coord *Chair's #: (717) 248-3933*	700 Pittt St Lewistown 17044			A	TCH	PBL	12	12	49	52	39	17
023	Lancaster Co Career and Tech Center Ms Wanda McGarvey, Coord *Chair's #: (717) 464-5070*	1730 Hans-Herr Dr Box 527 Willow Street 17584			A	TCH	PBL	12	12	85	118	98	0

School Code	Name of School, Director of Program, and Phone Number	Street Address / City or Town and Zip Code		Footnotes	Type of Program	NLNAC Accreditation as of January 31, 1998	Administrative Control	Financial Support (principal source)	Number of Months in Program	Educational Requirements for Entering Adult Program	Enrollments as of October 15, 1997	Admissions Aug. 1, 1996 - July 31, 1997	Graduations Aug. 1, 1996 - July 31, 1997	Fall Admissions Aug. 1, 1997 - Dec. 31, 1997
	PENNSYLVANIA													
	- Continued													
054	Lawrence County Area Voc-Tech Schoo Mrs Marlene Stoddard, Coord *Chair's #: (412) 654-2810*	750 Phelps Way	New Castle 16101			A	TCH	PBL	12	12	25	30	20	15
024	Lebanon Co Area Voc-Tech School Mrs Lynda Maurer, Supv *Chair's #: (717) 273-4401*	833 Metro Dr	Lebanon 17042			A	TCH	PBL	12	12	44	43	32	49
016	Lehigh Carbon Comm College Dr Doris L Branson, Coord *Chair's #: (610) 799-1547*	4525 Education Park Dr	Schnecksville 18078			A	CC	PBL	12	12	30	32	27	31
075	Lenape Area Voc-Tech School Ms Rebecca A Cappo, Coord *Chair's #: (412) 763-2608*	2215 Chaplin Ave	Ford City 16226			A	TCH	PBL	12	12	73	88	84	25
063	Mercer County Area Voc Tech Sch Ms Gloria Gill, Coord *Chair's #: (412) 662-3000 Ext 26*	776 Greenville Rd Box 152	Mercer 16137				TCH	PBL	120	12	63	65	45	0
076	Monroe Co Area Voc-Tech School Ms Sheila M Carolan, Coord *Chair's #: (717) 629-6563*	PO Box 66 Laurel Lake Dr	Bartonsville 18321			A	TCH	PBL	12	12	38	28	17	0
071	Northampton Comm Coll Ms Aurora Weaver, Dir *Chair's #: (610) 861-5376*	3835 Green Pond Rd	Bethlehem 18020		7		A	CC	PBL			Data reported w/AD prog			
080	Northern Tier Career Center Mrs Dorothy M Bennett, Coord *Chair's #: (717) 265-8113 Ext 25*	RR #1 Box 157A	Towanda 18848			A	TCH	PBL	12	12	23	19	14	24
036	PA College of Technology Mrs Linda Moran, Director *Chair's #: (717) 326-3761 Ext 4525*	One College Ave	Williamsport 17701				TCH	PBL	16	12	16	9	34	10
087	Parkway West Voc-Tech Sch Mrs Marion Mazzocco, Coord *Chair's #: (412) 923-1772 Ext 140*	7101 Steubenville Pike	Oakdale 15071			A	TCH	PBL			Publication withheld			
001	Pittsburgh Public Schs-Connelley Tech Dr Patricia Mashburn, Coord *Chair's #: (412) 338-3720*	1501 Bedford Ave	Pittsburgh 15219				TCH	PBL	12	12	48	86	94	30
015	Reading Area Comm College Mrs Merilee Grimes, Asst Dir *Chair's #: (610) 372-4721 Ext 5441*	10 S Second St PO Box 1706	Reading 19603			A	CC	PBL	12	12	36	45	33	38
022	Sch District of the City of Erie Miss Sheila M Warner, Coord *Chair's #: (814) 868-3345*	2931 Harvard Rd	Erie 16508			A	TCH	PBL	12	12	17	28	24	0

Explanation of footnotes on page x

School Code	Name of School, Director of Program, and Phone Number	Street Address / City or Town and Zip Code	Footnotes	Type of Program	NLNAC Accreditation as of January 31, 1998	Administrative Control	Financial Support (principal source)	Number of Months in Program	Educational Requirements for Entering Adult Program	Enrollments as of October 15, 1997	Admissions Aug. 1, 1996 - July 31, 1997	Graduations Aug. 1, 1996 - July 31, 1997	Fall Admissions Aug. 1, 1997 - Dec. 31, 1997
	PENNSYLVANIA												
	- Continued												
048	Schuylkill Training & Tech Center Ms Karen Runk, Dir *Chair's #: (717) 874-1034 Ext 131*	101 Technology Dr Frackville 17931			A	TCH	PBL			Publication withheld			
049	Somerset County Area Voc Tech School Ms Sibyl McNelly, Coord *Chair's #: (814) 445-8522*	6022 Glades Pike Suite 180 Somerset 15501			A	TCH	PBL	12	12	23	36	25	15
038	Univ of Pa-Prebysteriam Med Ctr Mrs Anna M Marshalick, Director *Chair's #: (215) 662-9161 Ext 9598*	39th St and Market Sts Philadelphia 19104			A	HSP	PVT			Publication withheld			
042	Upper Bucks Co Area Voc-Tech School Mrs Rachel Swierzewski, Supv *Chair's #: (215) 795-2234 Ext 224*	3115 Ridge Rd Perkasie 18944			A	TCH	PBL	12	12	44	42	35	44
047	Venango Co Area Voc-Tech Sch Mrs Sally Bowser, Coord *Chair's #: (814) 677-3097 Ext 207*	1 Voc-Tech Dr Oil City 16301			A	TCH	PVT	11	12	20	22	12	22
073	Warren County Area Voc-Tech School Mrs Carol A Goff, Coord *Chair's #: (814) 723-9290*	185 Hospital Dr Warren 16365			A	TCH	PBL	12	12	16	27	19	16
078	Western Area Career and Tech Center Mrs Nancy Lohr, Coord *Chair's #: (412) 746-2890 Ext 17*	688 Western Ave Canonsburg 15317			A	TCH	PBL	12	12	34	36	33	0
028	Westmoreland County Comm College Dr Patricia Milhalcin, Div Chair *Chair's #: (412) 925-4028*	Armbrust Rd Youngwood 15697	7			CC	PBL			Data reported w/AD prog			
026	Wilkes-Barre Area Voc Tech School Mrs Mary M Cawley, Coord *Chair's #: (717) 822-6539*	Box 1699 Jumper Rd Wilkes-Barre 18705			A	TCH	PBL	12	12	80	68	54	30
037	York County Area Voc-Tech School Ms Barbara Garzon, Admin *Chair's #: (717) 741-0820 Ext 256*	2179 S Queen St York 17402			A	TCH	PBL	11	12	57	66	53	34
	PUERTO RICO												
	42 Programs in 42 Schools												
023	Antilles Sch of Tech Careers Inc Mrs Carmen Ramirez, President *Chair's #: (787) 764-7576*	PO Box 1536 Hato Rey 00919			A	TCH	PVT	0	12	44	40	24	18
006	Antonio Luchetti Voc HS Ms Bedzaida Font, Coord *Chair's #: (787) 878-3130 Ext 30*	PO Box 601 Arecibo 00612				TCH	PBL			Publication withheld			

School Code	Name of School, Director of Program, and Phone Number	Street Address / City or Town and Zip Code	Footnotes	Type of Program	NLNAC Accreditation as of January 31, 1998	Administrative Control	Financial Support (principal source)	Number of Months in Program	Educational Requirements for Entering Adult Program	Enrollments as of October 15, 1997	Admissions Aug. 1, 1996 - July 31, 1997	Graduations Aug. 1, 1996 - July 31, 1997	Fall Admissions Aug. 1, 1997 - Dec. 31, 1997
	PUERTO RICO												
	- Continued												
026	Area Voc & Tech School-C F Daniels Mr Pagan Roche, Dir *Chair's #: (787) 762-7272*	Calle Jose Severo Quinones Carolina 00630				TCH	PBL			44	30	38	0
083	Atenas College Ms Maria Hernandez, Dir *Chair's #: (787) 884-3838*	PO Box 30160 Suite 146 Manati 00674				CC	PBL			Publication withheld			
008	Bernardino Cordero Voc HS Mrs Aida Torres De Lucca, Coord *Chair's #: (787) 842-7091 Ext 28*	Juan B Roman Ave Ponce 00731				TCH	PBL			Publication withheld			
062	Caribbean Educ & Training Corp Ms L Feliciano, Admin *Chair's #: (787) 250-1272*	America #411 Hato Rey 00919				TCH	PBL			Publication withheld			
032	Centro de Estudios Multidisciplinarios Miss Adriana Toledo, Dir *Chair's #: (787) 852-5505*	Vidal Dr #6 Humacao 00661				TCH	PVT			160	200	85	60
001	Centro de Estudios Multidisciplinarios Miss Adriana Toledo, Dir *Chair's #: (787) 765-4210 Ext 130*	602 Barbosa Ave Rio Piedras 00917				TCH	PVT			Publication withheld			
024	Colegio Tecnico de PR Ms Magali Estronga, Dir *Chair's #: (787) 856-7759*	Box 3020 Yauco 00698				CC	PBL			Publication withheld			
002	Columbia College Mrs Carmen Lopez, Coord *Chair's #: (787) 743-4041*	Carretera 183 KM 17 Caguas 00625	6			CC	PVT			Publication withheld			
047	D'Carmen Beauty & Tech Coll Ms Carmen Rodriguez, Dir *Chair's #: (787) 852-8655*	Box 38 Humacao 00791				CC	PVT			Publication withheld			
011	Dr Pedro Perea Voc HS Ms Gladys Hernandez, Director *Chair's #: (787) 833-0865*	PO Box 1330 Mayaguez 00681				TCH	PBL			73	30	33	0
009	Escuela Superior Vocacional Ms Melva A Gonzales, Director *Chair's #: (787) 890-2935*	PO Box 296 Ramey 00604				TCH	PBL			Publication withheld			
013	Escuela Tecnica Vocacional Mrs Rosa Vazquez, Dir *Chair's #: (787) 250-7502*	PO Box 150 Guayama 00654				TCH	PBL			Publication withheld			
004	Escuela Voc Metro Miguel Such Dr Teresa Brana-Ortega, Professor *Chair's #: (787 751-3780*	PO Box 21837 Upr Station Rio Piedras 00931		HS		GOV GOV	PBL PBL			Publication withheld			

Explanation of footnotes on page x

School Code	Name of School, Director of Program, and Phone Number	Street Address / City or Town and Zip Code	Footnotes	Type of Program	NLNAC Accreditation as of January 31, 1998	Administrative Control	Financial Support (principal source)	Number of Months in Program	Educational Requirements for Entering Adult Program	Enrollments as of October 15, 1997	Admissions Aug. 1, 1996 - July 31, 1997	Graduations Aug. 1, 1996 - July 31, 1997	Fall Admissions Aug. 1, 1997 - Dec. 31, 1997
	PUERTO RICO												
	- Continued												
037	Instituto de Banca y Comercio Ms Vivian Marrero, Counselor *Chair's #: (787) 854-6709*	Ave Munoz Rivera #996 Rio Piedras 00925				TCH	PVT			Publication withheld			
046	Instituto de Educacion Universal Mr Michael Santiago Sanchez, Dir *Chair's #: (809) 743-4747*	Calle Ruiz Belvis 52 Caguas 00725				TCH	PVT			Publication withheld			
035	Instituto de Educacion Universal Ms Blanca Robles, Coord *Chair's #: (809) 766-2435*	PO Box 209 Carolina 00628				TCH	PBL			Publication withheld			
044	Instituto Irma Valentin Ms Irma Valentin, President *Chair's #: (787) 894-1395*	Dr Cueto # 137 Utuado 00641				TCH	PBL	17	12	40	25	25	25
068	John Dewey College Dr Olga Desla, Director *Chair's #: (787) 753-0039*	Barbosa Ave #427 Hato Rey 00910				CC	PBL			First class in 1998			
022	Jose A Montanez Genaro Mrs Natividad Calderon, Professor *Chair's #: (787) 854-2250*	Carr 2 Km 47.3 PO Box 1091 Manati 00701				TCH	PBL			Publication withheld			
018	Jose N Gandara HS-Voc Prog Ms Nydia Perez Linares, Instructor *Chair's #: (787) 735-9072*	PO Box 1269 Aibonito 00609		HS		SEC SEC	PBL PBL	10 30	12 12	73 0	20 26	17 15	0 0
016	Luis Munoz Rivera HS Mrs Iris Martinez, Prof *Chair's #: (787) 894-2666*	Box 70 Utuado 00761				SEC	PBL			Publication withheld			
055	Metro College Mrs Rosa Julia Orama, Vice Pres *Chair's #: (787) 754-7120 Ext 223*	Ponce De Leon # 1126 San Juan 00925				TCH	PBL			Publication withheld			
049	Metro College Ms Geraldine Garcia, Dir *Chair's #: (787) 259-7272*	123 Calle Villa Ponce 00731				CC	PBL			Publication withheld			
057	National Coll of Business & Tech Ms Lourdes Balseiro, Dir *Chair's #: (787) 780-5134*	PO Box 2036 Bayamon 00960				TCH	PVT			Publication withheld			
056	National Coll of Business & Tech Mrs Maria Aleman, Millan, Dir *Chair's #: (809) 879-5045 Ext 243*	Gonzalo Marin #109 Arecibo 00612				TCH	PVT			Publication withheld			
085	Ponce Paramedical College Mr Leopoldo Vega, Director *Chair's #: (787) 848-1719*	Calle Acacia L-15 Ponce 00731				TCH	PBL			Publication withheld			

School Code	Name of School, Director of Program, and Phone Number	Street Address / City or Town and Zip Code		Footnotes	Type of Program	NLNAC Accreditation as of January 31, 1998	Administrative Control	Financial Support (principal source)	Number of Months in Program	Educational Requirements for Entering Adult Program	Enrollments as of October 15, 1997	Admissions Aug. 1, 1996 - July 31, 1997	Graduations Aug. 1, 1996 - July 31, 1997	Fall Admissions Aug. 1, 1997 - Dec. 31, 1997
	PUERTO RICO													
	- Continued													
027	Ponce Tech School Mrs Roxana Lanause, Director *Chair's #: (787) 844-7940*	Calle Salud #14 Ponce	00731				TCH	PBL			Publication withheld			
045	PR Tech & Beauty College Mr Angel Arriaga Rivera, Dir *Chair's #: (787) 785-3119*	Box 849 Bayamon	00621				CC	PBL			Publication withheld			
015	Republica de Costa Rica Voc HS Mrs Vilma Gracia, Nsg Teacher *Chair's #: (787) 743-4113*	PO Box 278 Caguas	00626				TCH	PBL			Publication withheld			
007	Ryder Memorial Hosp PN Program Mrs Sara Cruz Rivera, Dir *Chair's #: (787) 852-0768 Ext 4588*	PO Box 859 Humacao	00792			A	TCH	PVT	12	12	29	29	24	29
010	Santiago Veve HS-Dr Urgell Voc Prog Ms Hilda Collado Baez, Dir *Chair's #: (787) 863-0424*	Fajardo	00648		HS HSE		SEC SEC SEC	PBL PBL PBL	12 12	12 12 12	0 9	0 9	0 6	0 0
014	Thomas C Ongay Voc HS Mr German Figueroa , Interim Dir *Chair's #: (787) 785-3414*	PO Box 254 Bayamon	00956				SEC	PBL			Publication withheld			
063	Trinity College Ms Elizabeth Perez, Dir *Chair's #: (787) 842-0000 Ext 224*	Avenida Hostos 16 Ponce	00724				TCH	PVT			Publication withheld			
048	Universal Technology Coll of PR Inc Dr Raguel Batista, Dir *Chair's #: (787) 882-2065*	Calle Comercio Box 1955 Aguadilla	00605				TCH	PVT			Publication withheld			
	RHODE ISLAND													
	1 Program in 1 School													
001	Community College of Rhode Island Mrs Doris A Fournier, Chair *Chair's #: (401) 333-7217*	Louisquisset Pike Lincoln	02865	7		A	CC	PBL			Data reported w/AD prog			
	SOUTH CAROLINA													
	24 Programs in 24 Schools													
050	Aiken Technical College Mrs Ruth C Croom, Coordinator *Chair's #: (803) 593-9231 Ext 1404*	PO Drawer 696 Aiken	29802				TCH	PBL			Publication withheld			
024	Applied Technology Education Campus Mrs Sharon Clyburn, Coord *Chair's #: (803) 425-8982 Ext 48*	874 Vocational Lane Camden	29020				TCH	PBL			Publication withheld			
052	Central Carolina Tech Coll Mrs Laurie Harden, Dept Chair *Chair's #: (803) 778-7811*	506 North Guignard Dr Sumter	29150				TCH	PBL			Publication withheld			

Explanation of footnotes on page x

School Code	Name of School, Director of Program, and Phone Number	Street Address / City or Town and Zip Code		Footnotes	Type of Program	NLNAC Accreditation as of January 31, 1998	Administrative Control	Financial Support (principal source)	Number of Months in Program	Educational Requirements for Entering Adult Program	Enrollments as of October 15, 1997	Admissions Aug. 1, 1996 - July 31, 1997	Graduations Aug. 1, 1996 - July 31, 1997	Fall Admissions Aug. 1, 1997 - Dec. 31, 1997
	SOUTH CAROLINA													
	- Continued													
012	Cherokee Technology Center Mrs Janet Carroll, Coord *Chair's #: (864) 489-3191*	Box 3206 Cherokee Ave	Gaffney 29340		HSE		TCH TCH	PBL PBL	18 18	12 12	13 3	16 4	13 2	13 4
033	Chester Sch of PN Mrs Kathy Nance, Coord *Chair's #: (803) 377-1991*	121 Columbia St	Chester 29706				TCH	PBL	12	12	10	21	7	0
053	Chesterfield Marlboro Tech Coll Mrs Carolyn Wallace, Coord *Chair's #: (803) 921-6919 Ext 966*	PO Drawer 1007	Cheraw 29520				TCH	PBL		Publication withheld				
017	Conway Sch of PN Mrs Gail H Moss, Coord *Chair's #: (803) 365-5534 Ext 35*	335 Four Mile Rd	Conway 29526		HSE	A A	SEC SEC	PBL PBL	18	12	66 3	91 0	15 0	76 3
049	Florence Darlington Tech College Mrs Anne-Marie Goff, Dept Head *Chair's #: (803) 661-8180*	PO Box 100548	Florence 29501			A	TCH	PVT	12	12	11	22	10	0
004	Greenville Tech College Ms B Gayle Heller, Chair *Chair's #: (864) 250 8288*	PO Box 5616	Greenville 29606			A	TCH	PBL		Publication withheld				
018	Hartsville High Sch Mrs Athena Moree, Coord *Chair's #: (803) 383-3168*	701 Lewellyn Ave	Hartsville 29550				SEC	PBL	12	12	19	21	14	21
046	Horry-Georgetown Tech Coll PN Prog Mrs Mary Harper, Dept Head *Chair's #: (803) 546-8406*	4003 S Fraser St	Georgetown 29440				TCH	PBL		Publication withheld				
005	Lancaster Sch of PN Ms Denise Roberts, Coord *Chair's #: (803) 285-7404 Ext 238*	625 Normandy Rd	Lancaster 29720				TCH	PBL	12	12	18	18	14	18
025	Marion Sch of PN Mrs Mary L Pool, Coord *Chair's #: (803) 423-9800*	PO Box 890	Marion 29571		HSE		TCH TCH	PBL PBL	18 18	12 12	21 4	16 2	20 0	21 4
040	Midlands Technical College Ms Michelle Martin, Dir *Chair's #: (803) 822-3320*	PO Box 2408	Columbia 29202			A	TCH	PBL		Publication withheld				
047	Newberry County Career Ctr PN Prog Mrs Elaine Allacut, Coord *Chair's #: (803) 321-2674*	3413 Main St	Newberry 29108		HSE		SEC SEC	PBL PBL	18 9		16 3	14 3	12 3	10 3
028	Oconee Sch of PN-F P Hamilton Career Mrs Jane Finfrock, Coord *Chair's #: (864) 885-5011 Ext 28*	100 Vocational Dr	Seneca 29672		HSE		TCH TCH	PBL PBL	18		0 30	0 28	0 11	0 32

School Code	Name of School, Director of Program, and Phone Number	Street Address / City or Town and Zip Code	Footnotes	Type of Program	NLNAC Accreditation as of January 31, 1998	Administrative Control	Financial Support (principal source)	Number of Months in Program	Educational Requirements for Entering Adult Program	Enrollments as of October 15, 1997	Admissions Aug. 1, 1996 - July 31, 1997	Graduations Aug. 1, 1996 - July 31, 1997	Fall Admissions Aug. 1, 1997 - Dec. 31, 1997
	SOUTH CAROLINA												
	- Continued												
044	Orangeburg Calhoun Tech College Mrs Sandra Dewitt, Dept Head *Chair's #: (803) 535-1343*	3250 St Mathews Rd NE Orangeburg 29115			A	TCH	PBL	12	12	40	38	22	35
030	Piedmont Tech College Mrs Lena Warren, Dean *Chair's #: (864) 941-8536*	Emerald Rd, Drawer 1467 Greenwood 29646				TCH	PBL			Publication withheld			
001	Roper Hosp Mrs Beth Stone, Coord *Chair's #: (803) 763-2699*	316 Calhoun St Charleston 29401				HSP	PVT			Publication withheld			
013	Spartanburg Tech College Ms Linda Hayes, Dept Head *Chair's #: (864) 591-3868*	Drawer 4386 Spartanburg 29305				TCH	PBL	12	12	59	60	30	0
045	Tech College of the Lowcountry Dr R K Nunnery, Acting Dept Head *Chair's #: (803) 525-8267*	PO Box 1288 Beaufort 29902				TCH	PBL	12	12	28	30	22	29
014	Tri County Tech College Mrs Lynn M Lollis, Dept Head *Chair's #: (864) 261-1160*	PO Box 587 Pendleton 29670				TCH	PBL	12	12	26	20	18	25
051	Trident Tech College Mrs Alice Wieland, Dept Head *Chair's #: (803) 899-8021*	Box 118067 Charleston 29423				TCH	PBL	12	12	57	58	42	60
	SOUTH DAKOTA												
	2 Programs in 2 Schools												
004	Lake Area Tech Inst Mrs Julie Hanson, Dept Head *Chair's #: (605) 882-5284 Ext 286*	230 11th St NE Watertown 57201			A	TCH	PBL			34	34	27	34
006	Western Dakota Voc-Tech Inst Ms Donna Belitz, Coord *Chair's #: (605) 394-4034 Ext 112*	800 Michelson Dr Rapid City 57701				TCH	PBL	11	12	31	32	26	32
	TENNESSEE												
	26 Programs in 26 Schools												
021	Appalachian Reg PN Prog Mrs Annabelle Harvey, Coord *Chair's #: (615) 562-8648 Ext 33*	PO Box 419 Jackboro 37757				TCH	PBL			Publication withheld			
044	Baptist Memorial Coll Hlth Sciences Dr Veta Massey, Dean *Chair's #: (901) 227-6912*	1003 Monroe Ave Memphis 38104	1			COL	PVT			Publication withheld			
702	Blount Memorial Hosp Ms Polly Evans, Director *Chair's #: (423) 982 3134*	907 E Lamar Alexander Pky Maryville 37801				HSP	PVT	11	12	22	24	21	0

School Code	Name of School, Director of Program, and Phone Number	Street Address / City or Town and Zip Code	Footnotes	Type of Program	NLNAC Accreditation as of January 31, 1998	Administrative Control	Financial Support (principal source)	Number of Months in Program	Educational Requirements for Entering Adult Program	Enrollments as of October 15, 1997	Admissions Aug. 1, 1996 - July 31, 1997	Graduations Aug. 1, 1996 - July 31, 1997	Fall Admissions Aug. 1, 1997 - Dec. 31, 1997
	TENNESSEE												
	- Continued												
646	Bristol Program Mrs Barbara DeBusk, Director *Chair's #: (423) 652-9206*	Mcdowell St SlaterCenter Bristol City 37620				TCH	PBL	11	12	29	44	15	44
037	Chattanooga State Tech Comm College Mrs Donna Roddy, Dir *Chair's #: (423) 697-4447 Ext 4491*	4501 Amnicola Hwy Chattanooga 37406				CC	PBL	12	12	44	68	29	32
015	Columbia Nashville Memorial Hosp Mrs Anna House, Director *Chair's #: (615) 865-3578*	612 W Due West Ave Madison 37115				HSP	PVT			23	30	20	24
640	Four Rivers Regional PN Prog Mrs Belinda Douglas, Coord *Chair's #: (901) 475-2526 Ext 18*	PO Box 249 Covington 38019				TCH	PBL	12	12	43	52	67	20
022	Jackson Regional PN Program Ms Barbara Avent, Dir *Chair's #: (901) 424-0691 Ext 120*	2468 Westover Rd Jackson 38301				TCH	PBL	12	12	96	135	92	57
002	Methodist Hosp of PN Mrs Janie G Daniell, Dir *Chair's #: (901) 726-8861*	251 South Claybrook Memphis 38104				HSP	PVT	12	12	16	22	13	0
020	Metropolitan Nashville General Hosp Ms Carolyn Hunter, Dir *Chair's #: (615) 341-4283*	72 Hermitage Ave Nashville 37210	2			HSP	PBL			Publication withheld			
011	South Central Reg PN Ms Vicki Barnette, Dir *Chair's #: (615) 424-4014*	PO Box 614 Pulaski 38778	2			TCH	PBL			Publication withheld			
005	Sumner County PN Prog Mrs Cathy Eden Ammerman, Supv *Chair's #: (615) 452-4210 Ext 5164*	PO Box 1558 Gallatin 37066				SEC	PBL	11	12	21	24	18	24
038	TN Tech Center Mrs Anita Hemmeter, Supv *Chair's #: (423) 546-5567*	1100 Liberty St Knoxville 37919				TCH	PBL	12	12	51	60	44	33
034	TN Tech Center Mrs Sandra Wakefield, Dir *Chair's #: (615) 741-1241 Ext 34*	100 White Bridge Rd Nashville 37209				TCH	PBL			82	102	65	65
033	TN Tech Center Ms Roberta McCord, Director *Chair's #: (931) 473-5587 Ext 43*	241 Voc Tech Dr McMinnville 37110				TCH	PBL	12	12	10	16	8	0
031	TN Tech Center Mrs Terri Barnett Blevins, Dir *Chair's #: (615) 542-6656 Ext 25*	PO Box 789 1500 Arney St Elizabethton 37643				TCH	PBL			Publication withheld			

School Code	Name of School, Director of Program, and Phone Number	Street Address / City or Town and Zip Code		Footnotes	Type of Program	NLNAC Accreditation as of January 31, 1998	Administrative Control	Financial Support (principal source)	Number of Months in Program	Educational Requirements for Entering Adult Program	Enrollments as of October 15, 1997	Admissions Aug. 1, 1996 - July 31, 1997	Graduations Aug. 1, 1996 - July 31, 1997	Fall Admissions Aug. 1, 1997 - Dec. 31, 1997
	TENNESSEE													
	- Continued													
030	TN Tech Center Ms Terry Worley, Dir *Chair's #: (615) 441-6220*	740 Hwy 46 Dickson	37055				TCH	PBL			Publication withheld			
029	TN Tech Center Mrs Bonzella B Cook, Director *Chair's #: (931) 484-7502 Ext 38*	PO Box 2959 715 N Miller Ave Crossville	38555				TCH	PBL	12	12	31	24	23	25
028	TN Tech Center Mrs Linda Nein, Coord *Chair's #: (423)744-2814 Ext 215*	PO Box 848 Athens	37303				TCH	PBL	12	12	31	54	37	31
026	TN Tech Center Ms Linda Wier, Coord *Chair's #: (931) 685-5013 Ext 119*	1405 Madison Ave Shelbyville	37160				TCH	PBL	12	12	45	41	23	43
024	TN Tech Center Mrs Phyllis S Hime, Coord *Chair's #: (423) 586-5771 Ext 63*	821 W Louise St Box 130 Morristown	37813				TCH	PBL	12	12	75	95	60	45
023	TN Tech Center Ms Patrice Gilliam, Coord *Chair's #: (615) 823-5525 Ext 129*	PO Box 219 Livingston	38570				TCH	PBL			Publication withheld			
004	TN Tech Center Mrs Theresa Gillespie Isom, Coord *Chair's #: (901) 543-6126*	550 Alabama Ave Memphis	38105				TCH	PBL	12	12	18	51	35	0
025	TN Technology Center Ms Alice B McCutcheon, Coord *Chair's #: (901) 644-7365 Ext 37*	312 S Wilson St Paris	38242				TCH	PBL			36	25	37	31
008	Weakley Co Voc Center Mrs Gwendolyn Scarborough, Dir *Chair's #: (901) 364-5481*	8250 Hwy 22 Dresden	38225				TCH	PBL	11	12	23	24	20	12
	TEXAS													
	119 Programs in 71 Schools													
034	Alvin Comm College Ms Judy Siefert, Chair *Chair's #: (281) 388-4691*	3110 Mustang Rd Alvin	77511				CC	PBL	12	12	23	25	15	4
001	Amarillo College Mrs Sue McGee, Chair *Chair's #: (806) 354-6009*	Box 447 Amarillo	79178				CC	PBL			Publication withheld			
052	AMEDD Center School Dr Lynn Connelly, Chief Dept of Nsg *Chair's #: (210) 221-8336 Ext 8715*	2250 Stanley Rd MCCS-HNP Ft Sam Houston	78234		5			GOV	PBL			441	771	614	172

Explanation of footnotes on page x

Explanation of footnotes on page x

School Code	Name of School, Director of Program, and Phone Number	Street Address City or Town and Zip Code		Footnotes	Type of Program	NLNAC Accreditation as of January 31, 1998	Administrative Control	Financial Support (principal source)	Number of Months in Program	Educational Requirements for Entering Adult Program	Enrollments as of October 15, 1997	Admissions Aug. 1, 1996 - July 31, 1997	Graduations Aug. 1, 1996 - July 31, 1997	Fall Admissions Aug. 1, 1997 - Dec. 31, 1997
	TEXAS *- Continued*													
024	Angelina College Div of Hlth Careers Ms Jere Hammer, Coord *Chair's #: (409) 633-5265 Ext 241*	PO Box 1768 Lufkin	75901	7			CC	PBL			Data reported w/AD prog			
061	Austin Comm Coll Ms Yvonne VanDyke, Coord *Chair's #: (512) 223-6116*	PO Box 835 Fredericksburg	78624	1,7		A	CC	PBL			Publication withheld			
691	Austin Comm College Mrs Yvonne Vandyke, Dept Head *Chair's #: (512) 223-6116*	1020 Grove Austin	78741			A	CC	PBL	15	12	90	39	29	56
094	Baptist Hlth System Mrs Maxine Cadena, Director *Chair's #: (210) 302-2656*	511 Richmond Ave San Antonio	78205				HSP	PVT			Publication withheld			
030	Baptist Hlth System (Evening) Mrs Maxine Cadena, Director *Chair's #: (210)297-9100*	511 Richmond Ave San Antonio	78215				HSP	PVT			Publication withheld			
028	Bee Co College-Alice Extension Mrs Iva Burgan, Dir *Chair's #: (512) 664-1492*	704 Coyote Trail Alice	78332				CC	PBL			Publication withheld			
064	Bee Co College-Kingsville Branch Ms Noemi Arsona Peterson, Dir *Chair's #: (512) 593-2636*	PO Box 2140 Station I Kingsville	78363				CC	PBL			Publication withheld			
659	Bee County College Mrs Betty Sims, Dir *Chair's #: (512) 358-3130 Ext 2280*	3800 Charco Rd Beeville	78102				CC	PBL			Publication withheld			
756	Blinn College Ms Ina Eckert, Director *Chair's #: (409) 821-0202*	902 College Ave Brenham	77833				CC	PBL			18	18	15	18
762	Blinn College at Bryan Mrs Mary Arnold, Director *Chair's #: (409) 821-0203 Ext 38*	PO Box 6030 Bryan	77805	7			CC	PBL			Data reported w/AD prog			
604	Brazosport Comm College VN Prog Mrs Pamela Gwin, Dir *Chair's #: (409) 266-3290*	500 College Dr Lake Jackson	77566				CC	PBL	11	12	24	23	10	27
664	Central Texas College Dr Elaine E Hayes, Chair *Chair's #: (254) 526-1265*	6200 W Central TX Expresswa Killeen	76542				CC	PBL	12	12	75	94	68	12
783	Central Texas College-Brady Ext Dr Elaine E Hayes, Chair *Chair's #: (915) 597-2901 Ext 466*	Nine Rd Box 1361 Brady	76825				CC	PBL			Data with #664			

School Code	Name of School, Director of Program, and Phone Number	Street Address / City or Town and Zip Code	Footnotes	Type of Program	NLNAC Accreditation as of January 31, 1998	Administrative Control	Financial Support (principal source)	Number of Months in Program	Educational Requirements for Entering Adult Program	Enrollments as of October 15, 1997	Admissions Aug. 1, 1996 - July 31, 1997	Graduations Aug. 1, 1996 - July 31, 1997	Fall Admissions Aug. 1, 1997 - Dec. 31, 1997
	TEXAS												
	- Continued												
613	Cisco Jr College-Abilene Mrs Jackolyn Morgan, Dir Chair's #: (915) 673-4567 Ext 148	841 N Judge Ely Blvd Abilene 79601			A	CC	PBL			Publication withheld			
649	Clarendon College VN Program · Ms Vickie Moore, Dir Chair's #: (806) 874-3571 Ext 44	Box 968 Clarendon 79226	2			TCH	PBL			Publication withheld			
003	Del Mar College Mrs Bertha Almendarez, Chair Chair's #: (512) 886-1394	Baldwin & Ayers Corpus Christi 78404				CC	PBL			70	62	55	36
713	Delta Career Inst Voc Prog Mrs Charlotte Vannett, Director Chair's #: (409) 833-6161 Ext 411	1310 Pennsylvania Beaumont 77001				TCH	PVT	12	12	44	44	16	20
911	E & K Voc Nursing Prog Miss Paulette Potter, Dir Chair's #: (972) 630-6783	5415 Maple Ave Suite 114 Dallas 75235				TCH	PVT			Publication withheld			
652	El Centro College Ms Frances Warrick, Coord Chair's #: (214) 860-2288	Main & Lamar Dallas 75202			A	CC	PBL	12	12	38	42	32	19
006	El Paso Comm College Dr Paula R Mitchell, Div Chair Chair's #: (915) 831-4030	PO Box 20500 El Paso 79998	7	HSE		CC CC	PBL PBL			Data reported with/AD pro			
005	Extended Hlth Education Ms Gloria Edwards, Dir Chair's #: (817) 261-1594	1619 West Division Suite O Arlington 76012	2			TCH	PBL	12	12	24	24	19	24
070	Fort Duncan Medical Center Mrs Fe Sandoval, Dir Chair's #: (830) 773-5321 Ext 576	350 S Adams St Eagle Pass 78852				HSP	PBL			Publication withheld			
606	Frank Philips College-VN Prog Mrs Marilyn Wood, Chair Chair's #: (806) 274-5311 Ext 745	Box 5118 Borger 79008				TCH	PBL	12	12	55	76	49	0
665	Galveston Comm College Mrs Elizabeth Michel, Asst Dean Chair's #: (409) 763-6551 Ext 387	4015 Ave Q Galveston 77550				CC	PBL	12		21	28	19	22
639	Grayson County College Mrs Grace Cole, Dir Chair's #: (903) 786-4468	6101 Grayson Dr Denison 75021				CC	PBL	12	12	47	48	36	51
917	Health Care Training Center Mrs Maria Flecher, President Chair's #: (210) 687-8138	2715 Cornerstone Blvd Edinburg 78539	1			IND	PVT			8	0	8	10

Explanation of footnotes on page x

School Code	Name of School, Director of Program, and Phone Number	Street Address / City or Town and Zip Code	Footnotes	Type of Program	NLNAC Accreditation as of January 31, 1998	Administrative Control	Financial Support (principal source)	Number of Months in Program	Educational Requirements for Entering Adult Program	Enrollments as of October 15, 1997	Admissions Aug. 1, 1996 - July 31, 1997	Graduations Aug. 1, 1996 - July 31, 1997	Fall Admissions Aug. 1, 1997 - Dec. 31, 1997
	TEXAS — Continued												
089	Hill College Ms Sharon Allen, Dir Chair's #: (254) 582-2555 Ext 281	PO Box 619 Hillsboro 76645				CC	PBL	12	12	23	24	21	0
631	Hill College-Cleburne Ext Ms Paula Eubanks, Dir Chair's #: (817) 645-7522	1505 W Henderson Cleburne 76031				TCH	PBL			Publication withheld			
077	Hill College-Clifton Ms Helen M Amundson, Director Chair's #: (254) 675-6700	101 S Ave "T" Clifton 76634				TCH	PBL	12	12	12	12	12	12
021	Houston Comm College Ms Lucelia C Jones, Chair Chair's #: (713) 718-7332	3100 Shenandoah Houston 77021				CC	PBL	12	12	123	167	87	70
738	Howard College Mrs June Stone, Director Chair's #: (915) 264-5067	1001 Birdwell Ln Big Spring 79720				CC	PBL	12	12	18	22	15	18
012	Howard College-San Angelo Mrs Donna Rutledge, Dir Chair's #: (915) 947-9516 Ext 23	3197 Executive Dr San Angelo 76904	7	HSE		CC CC	PBL PBL	12 24	12 12	38 0	57 0	51 0	34 4
695	Jasper Mem Hosp Mrs Elizabeth Stovall, Dir Chair's #: (409) 384-1919 Ext 1868	1275 Marvin Hancock Dr Jasper 75951				HSP	PBL	12	10	16	16	15	16
653	Joe G Davis Sch of VN Mrs Barbara Bohanon, Director Chair's #: (409) 291-4544	3000 I-45 Huntsville 77340				HSP	PBL	12	12	17	19	17	19
638	John Peter Smith Sch Ms Loretta Mahaffey, Dir Chair's #: (817) 534-0200 Ext 116	1500 S Main St Fort Worth 76104				HSP	PBL	15	12	41	23	41	24
913	Kilgore College Mrs Barbara Brush, Dir Chair's #: (903) 753-2642	1100 Broadway Kilgore 75662				CC	PBL	12	12	51	70	21	32
774	Kilgore College-Longview Mrs Genie M Bartlett, Chair Chair's #: (903) 753-2642 Ext 24	300 S High St Longview 75601				CC	PBL			53	77	53	39
029	Kingwood College Mrs Thelma Bowie, Dir Chair's #: (281) 312-1647	20000 Kingwood Dr Kingwood 77339				CC	PBL	12	12	63	69	54	33
772	Lamar Univ at Orange Sch of Voc Nsg Mrs Sandra Dickey, Dir Chair's #: (409) 882-3311	410 Front St Orange 77630		HSE		CC CC	PBL PBL	12	12 12	84 0	96 0	72 0	48 0

School Code	Name of School, Director of Program, and Phone Number	Street Address / City or Town and Zip Code		Footnotes	Type of Program	NLNAC Accreditation as of January 31, 1998	Administrative Control	Financial Support (principal source)	Number of Months in Program	Educational Requirements for Entering Adult Program	Enrollments as of October 15, 1997	Admissions Aug. 1, 1996 - July 31, 1997	Graduations Aug. 1, 1996 - July 31, 1997	Fall Admissions Aug. 1, 1997 - Dec. 31, 1997
	TEXAS													
	- Continued													
010	Lamar Univ-Port Arthur Ext Ms Mary Mulliner, Coord *Chair's #: (409) 984-6362*	PO Box 310 Pt Arthur	77640				CC	PBL			92	96	84	45
614	Laredo Comm Coll Ms Dianna Miller, Dir *Chair's #: (210) 721-5255*	W End Washington St Laredo	78040				CC	PBL			Publication withheld			
755	Lee College Voc Nsg Prog Dr Rene Maher, Chair *Chair's #: (281) 425-6449 Ext 449*	PO Box 818 Baytown	77522				CC	PBL	12	12	37	40	32	40
097	McLennan Comm College (Career Ladd Mrs Alice Myers, Dir *Chair's #: (254) 299-8349*	1400 College Dr Waco	76708	7			CC	PBL			Data reported w/AD prog			
699	McLennan Comm College (Trad Prog) Mrs Leila Clark, Dir *Chair's #: (254) 299-8370*	1400 College Dr Waco	76708				CC	PBL			Publication withheld			
035	Memorial Hosp-Memorial City Sch of V Mrs Judith M Farmer, Director *Chair's #: (713) 932-3799*	920 Frostwood Houston	77024				HSP	PVT	12	12	39	47	24	0
692	Midland College Mrs Susan Jones, Dir *Chair's #: (915) 685-4600*	3600 N Garfield Midland	79701				CC	PBL	12	12	24	25	22	25
696	Midland College-Fort Stockton Ext Mrs Helen Dionne, Director *Chair's #: (915) 336-6541*	400 South Young Fort Stockton	79735				CC	PBL	12	12	15	15	3	15
915	Montgomery College Mrs Thelma Bowie, Dir *Chair's #: (281) 359-1683 Ext 1647*	2000 Kingwood Dr Kingwood	77339				CC	PBL	12	12	58	60	23	24
650	Navarro College Dr Judy Howden, Dir *Chair's #: (903) 874-6501 Ext 255*	Box 1170 Corsicana	75110				CC	PBL			Publication withheld			
082	Navarro College-Mexia Ext Dr Judy Howden, Director *Chair's #: (903) 874-6501*	PO Box 1132 Mexia	76667				CC	PBL			Publication withheld			
050	Navarro College-Waxahachie Ext Dr Judy Howden, Dir *Chair's #: (903) 874-6501 Ext 213*	1900 John Arden Dr Waxahachie	75165				CC	PBL	12	12	23	24	17	24
786	North Central TX College Ms Carol Brown, Dir *Chair's #: (817) 668-4291 Ext 291*	1525 W California Gainesville	76240				CC	PBL			75	130	82	110

Explanation of footnotes on page x

School Code	Name of School, Director of Program, and Phone Number	Street Address / City or Town and Zip Code		Footnotes	Type of Program	NLNAC Accreditation as of January 31, 1998	Administrative Control	Financial Support (principal source)	Number of Months in Program	Educational Requirements for Entering Adult Program	Enrollments as of October 15, 1997	Admissions Aug. 1, 1996 - July 31, 1997	Graduations Aug. 1, 1996 - July 31, 1997	Fall Admissions Aug. 1, 1997 - Dec. 31, 1997
	TEXAS													
	- Continued													
041	North Harris College Mrs Margaret Aalund, Director *Chair's #: (281) 618-5751*	2700 W W Thorne Dr Houston	77073	1,7			CC	PBL			Data reported w/AD prog			
720	Northeast TX Comm College Mrs Cynthia Amerson, Director *Chair's #: (903) 572-1911 Ext 356*	PO Box 1307 Mt Pleasant	75455				CC	PBL	12	12	36	36	24	37
711	Odessa College-Andrews Ext Ms Patricia Bayless, Dir *Chair's #: (915) 524-4022*	405 N W 3rd Andrews	79714				CC	PBL			Publication withheld			
725	Odessa College-Kermit Ext Mrs Anne Mitchell, Director *Chair's #: (915) 586-2369*	821 Jeffee Dr Kermit	79745				TCH	PBL			Publication withheld			
046	Odessa College-MEEP Dr Carol Boswell, Chair *Chair's #: (915) 335-6463*	201 W University Odessa	79760	7	HSE		CC CC	PBL PBL			Data reported w /AD prog			
909	Panola College Mrs Varonica Dickerson, Chair *Chair's #: (830) 694-4007*	PO Box 937 Marshall	95670				CC	PBL			Data with #769			
769	Panola College Mrs Varonica Dickerson, Chair *Chair's #: (903) 694-4007*	820 West Panola Carthage	75633				CC	PBL			Publication withheld			
059	Panola College Mrs Varonica Dickerson, Chair *Chair's #: (409) 598-2730*	PO Box 1863 Center	75935	1,7			CC	PBL			Data reported w\AD prog			
718	Paris Jr College (Ladder Prog) Mrs Virginia Holmes, Director *Chair's #: (903) 737-4355*	2400 Clarksville St Paris	75460	7			CC	PBL			Data reported w/AD prog			
698	Paris Jr College (Trad Voc Prog) Mrs Virginia Holmes, Dir *Chair's #: (903) 782-0734*	2400 Clarksville St Paris	75460				CC	PBL	14	12	56	84	78	58
905	Ranger College-Graham Ext Mrs Elaine Gates, Dir *Chair's #: (817) 549-4330*	Box 837 Graham	76046				CC	PBL			Publication withheld			
037	Ranger Jr College-Brownwood Ext Ms Kathy Brown, Dir *Chair's #: (915) 643-3852*	PO Box 837 Brownwood	76801				CC	PBL			Publication withheld			
090	San Jacinto Coll North Evening Mrs Serita Dickey, Chair *Chair's #: (281) 459-7114*	5800 Uvalde Houston	77049		HSE		CC CC	PBL PBL	12 12	12	62 0	75 0	55 0	71 0

School Code	Name of School, Director of Program, and Phone Number	Street Address, City or Town and Zip Code		Footnotes	Type of Program	NLNAC Accreditation as of January 31, 1998	Administrative Control	Financial Support (principal source)	Number of Months in Program	Educational Requirements for Entering Adult Program	Enrollments as of October 15, 1997	Admissions Aug. 1, 1996 - July 31, 1997	Graduations Aug. 1, 1996 - July 31, 1997	Fall Admissions Aug. 1, 1997 - Dec. 31, 1997
	TEXAS													
	- Continued													
038	San Jacinto College-North, Sch of VN Mrs Serita Dickey, Chair *Chair's #: (281) 459-7114*	5800 Uvalde Houston	77049	HSE			CC CC	PBL PBL			Publication withheld			
712	San Jacinto College-South Campus Mrs Joyce Pfleeger, Chair *Chair's #: (281) 922-3405*	13735 Beamer Rd Houston	77089				CC	PBL	12	12	83	109	63	52
708	Schreiner College VN Prog Mrs Rosemary Pullin, Director *Chair's #: (830) 792-2385*	Box 4491 Kerrville	78028				COL	PVT	12	12	48	52	53	30
741	South Plains College Mrs Marla K Cottenoir, Chair *Chair's #: (806) 894-9611 Ext 390*	1401 College Ave Levelland	79336				CC	PBL			Publication withheld			
704	South Plains College-Lubbock Ext Ms Barbara Bennett, Coord *Chair's #: (806) 747-0576 Ext 4622*	1302 Main Lubbock	79401				TCH	PBL			Publication withheld			
048	South Plains College-Plainview Ext Mrs Donna Womble, Director *Chair's #: (806) 291-4391*	708 Yonkers Plainview	79072				CC	PBL	12	12	34	36	27	36
916	South Texas Comm College Ms Melva Trevino, Chair *Chair's #: (956) 318-0101*	2524 N Closser Edinburg	78534				CC	PVT	0		35	35	26	35
914	Southwest Texas Jr College Mrs Suzanne Rue, Director *Chair's #: (830) 591-7316*	810 Bedell St Del Rio	78842				CC	PBL	9	12	18	18	14	17
728	Southwest Texas Jr College Mrs Suzanne Rue, Director *Chair's #: (830) 591-7316*	Box 70 Garner Field Rd Uvalde	78801				CC	PBL	12	12	34	35	22	34
022	St Philips College Ms Rebecca Hildebrand, Dir *Chair's #: (210) 531-3415*	1801 Martin Luther King San Antonio	78203	A			CC	PBL	11	12	166	178	153	87
658	St Philips College-New Braunfels Ext Mrs Susan Bell, Coord *Chair's #: (210) 606-9111 Ext 244*	610 N Houston St New Braunfels	78130				CC	PBL			Publication withheld			
743	Sul Ross Univ Mrs Judy Rayle, Dir *Chair's #: (915) 837-8171*	Box C-58 Alpine	79832				COL	PBL	12	12	9	12	10	9
700	Temple Jr College VN Prog Mrs Virginia Leak, Director *Chair's #: (254) 298-8666*	2600 S First Street Temple	76504				CC	PBL	12	12	55	43	43	0

Explanation of footnotes on page x

School Code	Name of School, Director of Program, and Phone Number	Street Address, City or Town and Zip Code	Footnotes	Type of Program	NLNAC Accreditation as of January 31, 1998	Administrative Control	Financial Support (principal source)	Number of Months in Program	Educational Requirements for Entering Adult Program	Enrollments as of October 15, 1997	Admissions Aug. 1, 1996 - July 31, 1997	Graduations Aug. 1, 1996 - July 31, 1997	Fall Admissions Aug. 1, 1997 - Dec. 31, 1997
	TEXAS *- Continued*												
092	Texarkana Comm College Mrs Carol Hodgson, Chair *Chair's #: (903) 838-4541 Ext 401*	2500 N Robinson Rd Box 9150 Texarkana 75501				CC	PBL	12	12	89	105	95	49
045	Texas Career Inc Ms Kiska Varela, Dir *Chair's #: (210) 308-8584 Ext 33*	1015 Jackson Keller San Antonio 78213	1			TCH	PBL	12	12	20	20	20	20
020	Texas State Tech Coll-Breckenridge Mrs Jackie Ververs, Coord *Chair's #: (915) 235-7388*	307 N Breckenridge Breckenridge 76424				TCH	PBL	12	12	13	12	10	14
075	Texas State Tech College Mrs Carrie Sanderson, Chair *Chair's #: (915) 235-7388 Ext 388*	Box 18 Rt3 Sweetwater 79556				TCH	PBL			Publication withheld			
910	The Health Inst of San Antonio Dr Peggy Richardson, Dir *Chair's #: (210) 733-3056*	6800 Park Ten Blvd Suite 160 San Antonio 78213				TCH	PVT			Publication withheld			
031	Tomball College Mrs Kathleen Emmite, Dir *Chair's #: (281) 357-3720*	30555 Tomball Parkway Tomball 77375	1,7			CC	PBL			Data reported w/AD prog			
908	Tri City Comm Hosp Sch of Voc Nsg Mrs Donna Zimmerman, Dir *Chair's #: (830) 769-3515 Ext 333*	Hwy 97 E PO Box 189 Jourdanton 78026				HSP	PVT	12	12	11	12	0	0
901	Trinity Valley Comm Coll Mrs Linda Bland, Coord *Chair's #: (903) 729-0256 Ext 29*	PO Box 2530 Palestine 75802				CC	PBL			Publication withheld			
095	Trinity Valley Comm College Mrs Helen Reid, Dean *Chair's #: (972) 932-4309*	800 Hwy 243 W Kaufman 75142				CC	PBL	12	12	56	53	42	33
752	Tyler County Hosp Mrs Eva Stanley, Director *Chair's #: (409) 283-8141 Ext 246*	1100 W Bluff Woodville 75979				HSP	PBL	12	12	15	15	15	0
004	Tyler Jr College Ms Jean Boyer, Dir *Chair's #: (903) 586-3000*	501 S S Ragsdale Jacksonville 75766				CC	PVT			Publication withheld			
017	Tyler Jr College VN Prog Ms Adelia Miller, Director *Chair's #: (903) 510-2470*	Box 9020 Tyler 75711				CC	PBL	12	10	58	60	51	60
084	Univ of Texas-Brownsville Ms Gloria Spencer, Dir *Chair's #: (956) 544-3865 Ext 1874*	80 Ft Brown Brownsville 78520				COL	PBL	12	12	50	48	45	24

Explanation of footnotes on page x

School Code	Name of School, Director of Program, and Phone Number	Street Address, City or Town and Zip Code	Footnotes	Type of Program	NLNAC Accreditation as of January 31, 1998	Administrative Control	Financial Support (principal source)	Number of Months in Program	Educational Requirements for Entering Adult Program	Enrollments as of October 15, 1997	Admissions Aug. 1, 1996 - July 31, 1997	Graduations Aug. 1, 1996 - July 31, 1997	Fall Admissions Aug. 1, 1997 - Dec. 31, 1997
	TEXAS												
	- Continued												
683	UTB-Texas Southmost College-Weslaco Ms Sally Roach, Director *Chair's #: (210) 956-5465*	PO Box 1110 Weslaco 78596				CC	PBL	12	10	43	36	27	48
715	Valley Baptist Medical Ctr Mrs Barbara Disbennett, Director *Chair's #: (210) 421-1721*	PO Drawer 2588 Harlingen 78550				HSP	PVT			Publication withheld			
912	Valley Grande Coll of Hlth and Technol Mrs Ramona Midamba, Director *Chair's #: (956) 973-1945 18*	800 W Railroad, Blgd W Box 8 Westasco 78596	HSE			IND IND	PVT PVT	17 17	12 12	97 2	54 2	34 4	56 0
018	Vernon Reg Jr College Ms Cathy J Bolton, Director *Chair's #: (817) 552-6291 Ext 270*	4400 College Dr Vernon 76384				CC	PBL			Publication withheld			
043	Vernon Reg Jr-Wichita Falls Miss Betty Duncan, Director *Chair's #: (940) 696-8752 Ext 3222*	4105 Maplewood Ave Wichita Falls 76308	HSE			CC CC	PBL PBL	12	12 12	123 0	130 0	68 0	66 0
757	Victoria College Ms Marilyn Powell, Coord *Chair's #: (512) 572-6446*	2200 East Red River St Victoria 77901				CC	PBL			177	180	143	192
015	Victoria College- Gonzales Mrs Faith Darilek, Director *Chair's #: (210) 672-7411*	1103 N Sarah Dewitt Dr Gonzales 78629				CC	PBL			Data with #757			
693	Victoria College-Cuero Ext Ms Deanna L Stenger, Director *Chair's #: (512) 275-6191 Ext 105*	2550 N Esplanade Cuero 77954				CC	PBL			Data with #757			
098	Victoria College-Port Lavaca Ext Mrs Madeline V Garcia, Director *Chair's #: (512) 552-8988*	810 N Ann St Port Lavaca 77979				CC	PBL			Data with #757			
902	Victoria College-Seguin Ext Mrs Gina Burns, Director *Chair's #: (210) 379-2411 Ext 397*	1331 East Court St Seguin 78155				CC	PBL			Data with #757			
074	Victoria College-Yoakum Comm Hosp Mrs Marilyn Morris, Director *Chair's #: (512) 573-3291 Ext 436*	303 Hubbard St, Box 753 Yoakum 77995				CC	PBL			Data with #757			
026	Victoria College-Zelda Allen Mrs Marianne Muehr, Director *Chair's #: (512) 798-2289*	1410 N Texana St Hallettsville 77964				CC	PBL			Data with #757			
025	Weatherford College VN Prog Mrs Katherine-Boswell, Director *Chair's #: (817) 594-5471 Ext 216*	308 E Park PO Box 5033 Weatherford 76086				CC	PBL			77	78	63	77

Explanation of footnotes on page x

School Code	Name of School, Director of Program, and Phone Number	Street Address / City or Town and Zip Code		Footnotes	Type of Program	NLNAC Accreditation as of January 31, 1998	Administrative Control	Financial Support (principal source)	Number of Months in Program	Educational Requirements for Entering Adult Program	Enrollments as of October 15, 1997	Admissions Aug. 1, 1996 - July 31, 1997	Graduations Aug. 1, 1996 - July 31, 1997	Fall Admissions Aug. 1, 1997 - Dec. 31, 1997
	TEXAS													
	- Continued													
609	Western Texas College-VN Prog Mrs Diane Beard, Director *Chair's #: (915) 573-8511 Ext 227*	College Ave Snyder	79549				CC	PBL			Publication withheld			
637	Wharton Co Jr Coll-Richmond Mrs Linda Herrera, Director *Chair's #: (281) 232-3775*	1601 Main Suite B-03 Richmond	77469				CC	PBL			33	36	18	36
019	Wharton Co Jr College Ms Nelta Maffett, Dir *Chair's #: (409) 532-6399*	911 Boling Highway Wharton	77488				CC	PBL			45	26	29	26
603	Wharton Co Jr College-Bay City Mrs Nelta Maffett, Dir *Chair's #: (409) 532-6491*	911 E Boling Wharton	77488				CC	PBL			Publication withheld			
	UTAH													
	7 Programs in 8 Schools													
007	Coll of Eastern Utah at Price Ms Diana Baker, Dir *Chair's #: (435) 637-2120 Ext 5261*	451 E 400, N Price	84501				CC	PBL	9	12	50	32	26	50
004	Dixie College Mr Kevin Tipton, Dir *Chair's #: (435) 652-7863*	225 S 700 E St George	84770	2			CC	PBL	10	12	21	28	28	21
002	Salt Lake Community College Ms Marilyn Little, Coord *Chair's #: (801) 957-5704*	4600 S Redwood Rd Box 3080 Salt Lake City	84130	7		A	CC	PBL			Data reported w/AD prog			
010	Sevier Valley Applied Tech Center Susan Ferguson, Director *Chair's #: (801) 896-9729*	800 W 200 South Richfield	84701				TCH	PBL			Publication withheld			
009	Uintah Basin Area Tech Ctr Mr Brett Robbins, Director *Chair's #: (801) 722-4523 Ext 114*	1100 E Lagoon St PO 124-5 Roosevelt	84066				TCH	PBL			Publication withheld			
001	Utah Valley State College Mrs Karin L Swendsen, Director *Chair's #: (801) 222-8190*	800 West 1200 South Orem	84058				COL	PBL			Publication withheld			
005	Weber State University Dr Karen W Beaver, Coord *Chair's #: (801) 626-6737*	3750 Harrison Blvd Ogden	84408	7		A	COL	PBL	12	12	35	49	45	49
	VERMONT													
	4 Programs in 1 School													
003	Vermont Tech College Ms Patricia Menchini, Dir *Chair's #: (802) 655-2540*	29 Ethan Allen Ave Colchester	05446			A	TCH	PBL			Data with #001			

School Code	Name of School, Director of Program, and Phone Number	Street Address / City or Town and Zip Code	Footnotes	Type of Program	NLNAC Accreditation as of January 31, 1998	Administrative Control	Financial Support (principal source)	Number of Months in Program	Educational Requirements for Entering Adult Program	Enrollments as of October 15, 1997	Admissions Aug. 1, 1996 - July 31, 1997	Graduations Aug. 1, 1996 - July 31, 1997	Fall Admissions Aug. 1, 1997 - Dec. 31, 1997
	VERMONT												
	- Continued												
001	Vermont Tech College Ms Patricia Menchini, Dir Chair's #: (802) 447-5419	Bennington 05201			A	TCH	PBL	11	12	93	98	83	121
006	Vermont Technical College Ms Patricia Menchini, Dir Chair's #: (802) 728-1341	PO Box 500 Randolph Center 05061			A	TCH	PBL	Data with #001					
002	Vermont Technical College Ms Patricia Menchini, Dir Chair's #: (802) 254-5570	30 Maple St Brattleboro 05301	'		A	TCH	PBL	Data with #001					
	VIRGIN ISLANDS												
	1 Program in 1 School												
900	St Croix Voc Skill Center Mrs Cynthia Vanwingerden, Coord Chair's #: (340) 778-2216 Ext 234	21 22 & 23 Hospital St Christiansted St 00820	HSE			TCH TCH	PBL PBL	14 24	12 12	11 31	11 31	8 22	11 15
	VIRGINIA												
	63 Programs in 56 Schools												
055	Alexandria City Schs / Alex Hosp Ms Sandra Ballif, Director Chair's #: (703) 824-6800 Ext 6858	3330 King St Alexandria 22302	HSE			SEC SEC	PBL PBL	18 18	12	29 14	35 7	28 4	33 18
037	Bedford County Schs-Mem Hosp Mrs Carolyn Roaf, Dir Chair's #: (540) 587-5493	1613 Oakwood St Bedford 24523	HSE			SEC SEC	PBL PBL	18	12	0 25	0 15	0 11	0 15
040	Buchanan County Sch Mrs Sandra Cook, Director Chair's #: (540) 935-4541	Rt 5 Box 110 Grundy 24614	HSE			SEC SEC	PBL PBL	Publication withheld					
015	Carilion Roanoke Mem Hosp Sch Mrs Carolyn W Lyon, Director Chair's #: (540) 981-7362	PO Box 13367 Roanoke 24033				HSP	PVT	12	12	23	25	21	26
074	Centra Hlth School of PN Mrs Patricia Uzsoy, Dean Chair's #: (804) 947-3070 Ext 3070	1901 Tate Springs Rd Lynchburg 24503			A	HSP	PVT	16	12	28	15	10	15
052	Central Sch-Norfolk Tech-Voc Center Miss Gloria Rudibaugh, Prog Leader Chair's #: (757) 441-5625	1330 N Military Hwy Norfolk 23502	HSE		A A	SEC SEC	PBL PBL	18		18 44	10 27	6 12	10 33
012	Charlottesvl-Albemrl-M Jefferson Hosp Ms Bonita Howard, Coord Chair's #: (804) 973-4461	1000 E Rio Road Charlottesvil 22901	HSE			TCH TCH	PBL PBL	18	12	7 4	19 1	16 0	7 4
048	Chesapeake Tech Ctr Sch of PN Mrs Kathleen A Jones, Director Chair's #: (757) 547-0134	1617 Cedar Rd Chesapeake 23320				SEC	PBL	Publication withheld					

Explanation of footnotes on page x

School Code	Name of School, Director of Program, and Phone Number	Street Address, City or Town and Zip Code		Footnotes	Type of Program	NLNAC Accreditation as of January 31, 1998	Administrative Control	Financial Support (principal source)	Number of Months in Program	Educational Requirements for Entering Adult Program	Enrollments as of October 15, 1997	Admissions Aug. 1, 1996 - July 31, 1997	Graduations Aug. 1, 1996 - July 31, 1997	Fall Admissions Aug. 1, 1997 - Dec. 31, 1997
	VIRGINIA													
	- Continued													
067	Chesterfield Co Pub Schs Mrs Sandra Foote, Director *Chair's #: (804) 768-6160*	10101 Courthouse Rd Chesterfield	23832		HSE		SEC SEC	PBL PBL	18 18	12 12	42 14	28 14	18 0	20 20
019	Commonwealth Tech Institute Ms Evelyn Stone, Dir *Chair's #: (757) 467-2153*	5265 Providence Rd Virginia Beach	23464	2			TCH	PVT			Publication withheld			
078	Computer Dynamics Inst, Inc Ms Kathleen Shovelin, Prog Manager *Chair's #: (757) 499-4900 Ext 31*	5361 Virginia Beach Blvd Virginia Beach	23462				TCH	PVT			Publication withheld			
038	Dabney S Lancaster Comm Coll Ms Lisa Allison-Jones. Head *Chair's #: 9540) 863-2843*	PO Box 1000 Clifton Forge	24422	2			CC	PBL			Publication withheld			
011	Danville Comm College Mrs Lajuana Jordan, Director *Chair's #: (804) 791-5356*	1008 S Main St Danville	24541				CC	PBL	12	12	22	40	18	29
024	Fairfax Co School of PN Mrs Patricia Nelsen, Coord *Chair's #: (703) 207-4011 Ext 4092*	7423 Camp Alger Ave Falls Church	22042		HSE		SEC SEC	PBL PBL	9	12	34 39	18 56	21 24	37 40
013	Fredericksburg Area Sch of PN Mrs Sandra Demotses, Director *Chair's #: (540) 891-0675*	6713 Smith Station Rd Spotsylvania	22553		HSE		SEC SEC	PBL PBL	20	12	28 14	12 18	16 0	13 16
021	G Washington Carver-Piedmont Educ Ct Mrs Esther Frazier-Petty, Dir *Chair's #: (540) 825-0476 Ext 8*	PO Box 999 Culpeper	22701		HSE		TCH TCH	PBL PBL	18 18	12 12	32 2	16 1	16 1	17 1
050	Giles County Tech Center Mrs Nancy B Dowdy, Director *Chair's #: (540) 921-1166 Ext 0016*	PO Box 479 Pearisburg	24134		HSE		SEC SEC	PBL PBL	18 .	12 12	10 13	16 0	0 4	12 14
045	Greensville County Schs-Mem Hosp Mrs Ann W Wrenn, Director *Chair's #: (804) 634-4294*	403 Harding St Emporia	23847		HSE		TCH TCH	PBL PBL			Publication withheld			
042	Henrico Co Schools-St Mary's Hospital Ms Ann L Unholz, Director *Chair's #: (804) 328-4095*	201 E Nine Mile Rd Highland Springs	23075		HSE	A A	SEC SEC	PBL PBL	18	12	0 33	0 62	0 36	0 65
035	Henry Co Schs-Memorial Hosp Mrs Rebecca Greer, Dir *Chair's #: (540) 656-0271*	PO Box 5311 Martinsville	24115		HSE		SEC SEC	PBL PBL	18	12	57 6	20 9	25 3	26 6
062	Lafayette Sch of PN Mrs Karen Spangler, Coord *Chair's #: (757) 565-4270*	4460 Longhill Rd Williamsburg	23188		HSE		SEC SEC	PBL PBL			Publication withheld			

Explanation of footnotes on page x

School Code	Name of School, Director of Program, and Phone Number	Street Address / City or Town and Zip Code	Footnotes	Type of Program	NLNAC Accreditation as of January 31, 1998	Administrative Control	Financial Support (principal source)	Number of Months in Program	Educational Requirements for Entering Adult Program	Enrollments as of October 15, 1997	Admissions Aug. 1, 1996 - July 31, 1997	Graduations Aug. 1, 1996 - July 31, 1997	Fall Admissions Aug. 1, 1997 - Dec. 31, 1997
	VIRGINIA												
	- Continued												
053	Lee County Voc Tech Sch / Mrs Julia C Wyrick, Director / *Chair's #: (540) 346-1960*	One Vo Tech Dr Box 100 / Ben Hur 24218		HSE		SEC / SEC	PBL / PBL			Publication withheld			
005	Lord Fairfax Comm Coll / Ms Betty Ward, Dir / *Chair's #: (540) 722-3458*	156 Dowell J Circle / Winchester 22602				CC	PBL	12	12	48	47	16	45
064	Loudoun Co Pub Schs-C Monroe V-T C / Mrs Karen E Mason, Director / *Chair's #: (703) 771-6560*	715 Childrens Ctr Rd SW / Leesburg 20175		HSE		TCH / TCH	PBL / PBL	18 / 18	12 / 12	34 / 7	21 / 5	14 / 0	19 / 6
059	Massanutten Tech Center / Ms Linda Wood, Supv / *Chair's #: (540) 434-5961 Ext 128*	325 Pleasant Valley Rd / Harrisonburg 22801		HSE		TCH / TCH	PBL / PBL	/ 18	/ 12	44 / 5	34 / 3	17 / 1	24 / 5
070	Medical Careers Inst / Mrs Barbara Ellington, Dir / *Chair's #: (757) 873-2423*	605 Thimble Shoals Blvd / Newport News 23606				IND	PVT			Publication withheld			
009	MedTech Hlth Care Training / To be named / *Chair's #: (703) 360-3848*	8794 Sacramento Dr / Alexandria 22309	2			TCH	PBL			Publication withheld			
010	New Horizon Reg Educ Center / Mrs Mary S Armstead, Coord / *Chair's #: (757) 766-1291*	520 Butler Farm Rd / Hampton 23666			A	TCH	PBL	0	12	0	0	0	0
025	New River Comm College / Mrs LaRue Ridenhour, Asst Prof / *Chair's #: (540) 674-3600 Ext 251*	PO Box 1127 / Dublin 24084				CC	PBL	12	12	25	30	16	30
014	Northampton-Accomack County Schs / Mrs Bonnie R Nordstrom, Director / *Chair's #: (757) 442-8771*	PO Box 17 10098 Rogers Dr / Nassawadox 23413				TCH	PBL	12	12	15	17	12	13
029	Page County Tech Center / Mrs Jessica Ressler, Dir / *Chair's #: (540) 778-4276*	525 Middleburg Rd / Luray 22835	2	HSE		TCH / TCH	PBL / PBL	/ 18		0 / 10	0 / 10	0 / 10	0 / 10
016	Petersburg City Schs-Southside Reg / Mrs Jean Riddle, Coord / *Chair's #: (804) 862-7078*	816 E Bank St / Petersburg 23803		HSE		SEC / SEC	PBL / PBL			Publication withheld			
044	Portsmouth Public Sch of PN / Mrs Katherine B Decker, Director / *Chair's #: (757) 393-5408*	3701 Willett Dr / Portsmouth 23707		HSE		TCH / TCH	PBL / PBL			Publication withheld			
001	Prince William Co Schs / Mrs Bette Sneed, Dir / *Chair's #: (703) 791-7357*	PO Box 389 / Manassas 20108		HSE		SEC / SEC	PBL / PBL	/ 18	/ 12	0 / 66	0 / 47	0 / 26	0 / 0

School Code	Name of School, Director of Program, and Phone Number	Street Address / City or Town and Zip Code		Footnotes	Type of Program	NLNAC Accreditation as of January 31, 1998	Administrative Control	Financial Support (principal source)	Number of Months in Program	Educational Requirements for Entering Adult Program	Enrollments as of October 15, 1997	Admissions Aug. 1, 1996 - July 31, 1997	Graduations Aug. 1, 1996 - July 31, 1997	Fall Admissions Aug. 1, 1997 - Dec. 31, 1997
	VIRGINIA													
	- Continued													
058	Radford City PN Sch Mrs Virginia Graham Jones, Dir *Chair's #: (540) 731-2678*	PO Box 3698 Radford	24143		HS		SEC SEC	PBL PBL	 12		0 36	16 7	0 17	0 24
071	Rappahannock Comm College Mrs Dianne Lucy, Prog Head *Chair's #: (804) 758-6779*	12745 College Dr Glenns	23149				CC	PBL	12	12	30	35	23	30
043	Richmond Public Schools Ms Hilda Roundtree, Specialist *Chair's #: (804) 780-6076*	2020 Westwood Ave Richmond	23230		HSE	A A	TCH TCH	PBL PBL			Publication withheld			
027	Riverside Hlth System & Newpt News S Mrs Brenda Booth, Coord *Chair's #: (757) 594-2720*	12420 Warwick Blvd Newport News	23606		HSE	A A	SEC SEC	PBL PBL	11 20	12 12	33 16	33 11	21 1	34 16
004	Russell Co Voc Sch of PN Mrs Kimberley Israel, Dir *Chair's #: (540) 889-6547*	1 Vocational Sch Rd Box 849 Lebanon	24266		HSE		TCH TCH	PBL PBL			Publication withheld			
079	Salem Sch of PN Mrs Martha Barnas, Prog Head *Chair's #: (540) 847-6283*	400 N Spartan Dr Salem	24153		HSE		CC CC	PBL PBL			Publication withheld			
030	Scott Co Voc Center Mrs Brigitte Casteel, Dir *Chair's #: (540) 386-6515*	150 Broadwater Gate City	24251	2	HSE		TCH TCH	PBL PBL	18 18	12 12	45 4	25 4	15 4	26 4
041	Smyth County Voc Sch of PN Ms Georgia Miller, Dir *Chair's #: (540) 646-8117*	Rt 2 Box 653 Marion	24354		HSE		TCH TCH	PBL PBL	 18	 12	0 34	0 23	0 13	0 20
033	Southampton Mem Hosp Mrs Ercelle Vann, Dir *Chair's #: (757) 569-6414*	100 Fairview Dr Franklin	23851				HSP	PBL	12	12	15	15	12	15
046	Southside Sch of PN Mrs Pamela Fowler, Dir *Chair's #: (804) 315-2630*	800 Oak Street Farmville	23901				TCH	PBL	12	12	20	20	19	0
073	Southside VA Comm College Ms Shirley Bugg, Prof *Chair's #: (804) 949-1037*	109 Campus Dr Alberta	23821				CC	PBL			Publication withheld			
002	Southside VA Comm College Mrs Annie Lee Owen, Dir *Chair's #: (804) 575-3100 Ext 320*	2204 Wilborn Ave South Boston	24592				CC	PBL			Publication withheld			
034	Stonewall Jackson Hosp Mrs Penny Fauber-Moore, Director *Chair's #: (540) 462-1351*	One Health Circle Lexington	24450				SEC	PBL	11	12	13	15	9	0

Explanation of footnotes on page x

School Code	Name of School, Director of Program, and Phone Number	Street Address / City or Town and Zip Code	Footnotes	Type of Program	NLNAC Accreditation as of January 31, 1998	Administrative Control	Financial Support (principal source)	Number of Months in Program	Educational Requirements for Entering Adult Program	Enrollments as of October 15, 1997	Admissions Aug. 1, 1996 - July 31, 1997	Graduations Aug. 1, 1996 - July 31, 1997	Fall Admissions Aug. 1, 1997 - Dec. 31, 1997
	VIRGINIA												
	- Continued												
020	Suffolk Public Sch-Obici Mem Hosp Ms Gwen T Sweat, Director *Chair's #: (757) 934-4826*	Louise Obici Mem Hosp Box 1 Suffolk 23439			A	HSP	PBL	12	12	17	25	13	0
003	Tazewell Co Career Tech Center Ms Dolores Mulkey, Director *Chair's #: (540) 596-6650*	114 Maplewood Ln Tazewell 24651	HSE		A A	TCH TCH	PBL PBL	18	12	0 41	0 34	0 21	0 34
068	Twin Co Sch of PN/WCC Mr Jeffrey Miller, Prog Head *Chair's #: (540) 238-1177*	121 W Grayson St Galax 24333	HSE			CC CC	PBL PBL			Publication withheld			
006	Valley Voc-Tech Ctr Sch of Nsg Mrs G G Hildebrand, Director *Chair's #: (540) 245-5002*	Rt 3 Box 265 Fisherville 22939				TCH	PBL			Publication withheld			
060	Virginia Beach Sch of PN Ms Rose Mary Saliba, Director *Chair's #: (757) 427-5300*	2925 N Landing Rd Virginia Beach 23456	HSE		A A	TCH TCH	PBL PBL	24	12 12	36 54	27 36	15 20	21 39
049	Virginia Western Comm Coll Ms Martha Barnas, Prog Head *Chair's #: (540) 857-6283*	Po Box 14007 Roanoke 24038	2 HS			CC CC	PBL PBL			Publication withheld			
054	Washington County Schs Mrs Margaret B Humphreys, Dir *Chair's #: (540) 628-1870*	255 Stanley St Abingdon 24210	HSE			TCH TCH	PBL PBL	18 9	12 12	32 5	21 7	9 4	17 5
018	Wise County Voc Tech Sch of PN Ms Jennifer Hall, Dir *Chair's #: (540) 328-6113*	PO Box 1218 Wise 24293				SEC	PBL			Publication withheld			
	WASHINGTON												
	25 Programs in 23 Schools												
015	Bellingham Tech Coll Ms Ruby Mans, Coordinator *Chair's #: (360) 738-3105 Ext 432*	3028 Lindbergh Ave Bellingham 98225				TCH	PBL	15	12	87	89	35	36
026	Big Bend Comm College Mrs Linda Wrynn, Dir *Chair's #: (509) 762-6285 Ext 285*	Moses Lake 98837				CC	PBL	11	12	13	15	12	14
011	Centralia College Mrs Gail J Wrzesinski, Dir *Chair's #: (360) 736-9391 Ext 252*	600 West Locust Centralia 98531				CC	PBL	12	12	26	25	25	26
007	Clark College Ms Linda E Hein, Director *Chair's #: (360) 992-2192*	1800 E McLoughlin Blvd Vancouver 98663				TCH	PBL	12	12	20	29	19	20

Explanation of footnotes on page x

School Code	Name of School, Director of Program, and Phone Number	Street Address, City or Town and Zip Code	Footnotes	Type of Program	NLNAC Accreditation as of January 31, 1998	Administrative Control	Financial Support (principal source)	Number of Months in Program	Educational Requirements for Entering Adult Program	Enrollments as of October 15, 1997	Admissions Aug. 1, 1996 - July 31, 1997	Graduations Aug. 1, 1996 - July 31, 1997	Fall Admissions Aug. 1, 1997 - Dec. 31, 1997
	WASHINGTON - Continued												
021	Clover Park Tech Coll Mrs Sheila Reilly, Dir Chair's #: (253) 589-5536	4500 Steilacoom Blvd, SW Lakewood Center 98499				TCH	PBL			Publication withheld			
013	Columbia Basin College Ms Donna E Campbell, Dean Chair's #: (509) 547-0511 Ext 283	2600 N 20th Pasco 99301	7			CC	PBL			Data reported w/AD prog			
005	Everett Community College Mr Stuart Barger, Director Chair's #: (425) 388-9399	801 Wetmore Ave Everett 98201	7			CC	PBL			Data reported w/AD prog			
010	Grays Harbor Coll Dr Candice Mohar, Chair Chair's #: (360) 538-4148	1620 Edwards Smith Dr Aberdeen 98520	1			CC	PBL			Publication withheld			
027	Green River Comm College Ms Julia Short, Coordinator Chair's #: (206) 833-9111	12401 SE 320th St Auburn 98002				CC	PBL			Publication withheld			
003	L H Bates Technical College Mr Jeffrey Bonnell, Dir Chair's #: (253) 596-1617	1101 S Yakima Tacoma 98405				TCH	PBL	15	12	60	95	60	49
037	Lake Washington Tech College Ms Patricia Stuart, Coord Chair's #: (206) 828-5600	11605 132nd Ave NE Kirkland 98034	7			TCH	PBL			Data reported w/AD prog			
014	Lower Columbia College Ms Helen Hing, Director Chair's #: (360) 577-3446	1600 Maple Longview 98632	7			CC	PBL			Data reported w/AD Prog			
030	North Seattle Comm College Ms Sandra Liming, Coord Chair's #: (206) 527-3791	9600 College-Way, N Seattle 98103				CC	PBL	12	12	74	49	24	44
034	Oak Harbor PN Prog-Skagit Valley Coll Ms Kathleen A Petet, Dept Chair Chair's #: (360) 679-5324	1900 SE Pioneer Way Oak Harbor 98277				CC	PBL	11	12	32	37	31	32
004	Olympic College Mrs Marge Herzog, Coord Chair's #: (360) 478-4604	1600 Chester Ave Bremerton 98310	7			CC	PBL			Data reported w/AD Prog			
036	Renton Technical College Ms Toni Whitefield, Assoc Dean Chair's #: (206) 383-2352 Ext 5552	3000 NE 4th St Renton 98056				TCH	PBL	11	12	53	67	41	35
012	Skagit Valley College Mrs Flora G Adams, Chair Chair's #: (360) 416-7631	2405 College Way Mount Vernon 98273	7			CC	PBL			Data reported w/AD prog			

Explanation of footnotes on page x

School Code	Name of School, Director of Program, and Phone Number	Street Address / City or Town and Zip Code	Footnotes	Type of Program	NLNAC Accreditation as of January 31, 1998	Administrative Control	Financial Support (principal source)	Number of Months in Program	Educational Requirements for Entering Adult Program	Enrollments as of October 15, 1997	Admissions Aug. 1, 1996 - July 31, 1997	Graduations Aug. 1, 1996 - July 31, 1997	Fall Admissions Aug. 1, 1997 - Dec. 31, 1997
	WASHINGTON												
	- Continued												
032	South Puget Sound Comm College Ms Ruby Flesner, Director *Chair's #: (360) 754-7711 Ext 285*	2011 Mottman Rd, SW Olympia 98502				CC	PBL	11	12	23	24	23	23
002	Spokane Comm Coll Mrs Carol Nelson, Dir *Chair's #: (509) 533-7311*	N 1810 Greene St Spokane 99207				CC	PBL	15		0	39	0	32
017	Walla Walla Comm College (2 Branches) Mrs Marilyn Galusha, Dir *Chair's #: (509) 527-4240*	500 Tausick Way Walla Walla 99362	7			CC	PBL			Data reported w/AD prog			
008	Wenatchee Valley College Ms Connie Barnes, Dir *Chair's #: (509) 664-2532*	1300 5th St Wenatchee 98801	7			CC	PBL			Data reported w/AD prog			
035	Wenatchee Vly College-Omak Branch Mrs Connie Barnes, Director *Chair's #: (509) 665-2605*	1300 So 5th Wenatchee 98801	7			CC	PBL			Data reported w/AD prog			
006	Yakima Valley College (3 Branches) Dr Bronwynne Evans, Dept Head *Chair's #: (509) 574-4902*	PO Box 1647 Yakima 98907	7			CC	PBL			Data reported w /AD prog			
	WEST VIRGINIA												
	21 Programs in 21 Schools												
006	Academy Career Technology Ms Ella Pennington, Coord *Chair's #: (304) 256-4675*	390 Stanaford Rd Beckley 25801				TCH	PBL	12		34	39	33	35
001	B M Spurr Sch of Practical Nursing Mrs Carol Storm, Director *Chair's #: (304) 232-8814*	800 Wheeling Ave Glen Dale 26038			A	HSP	PVT	12	12	18	19	17	18
005	Cabell Co Voc-Tech Ctr Mrs Patricia Bailey, Chair *Chair's #: (304) 528-5108*	1035 Norway Ave Huntington 25705				TCH	PBL			Publication withheld			
016	Fayette Co Sch of PN Mrs Sandra Wriston, Coord *Chair's #: (304) 442-4222*	Box 459 Smithers 25186				SEC	PBL	11	12	22	22	21	22
027	Fred W Eberle School of Practical Nsg Mrs Deborah Carpenter, Coord *Chair's #: (304) 472-1276 Ext 111*	Rt 5 Box 2 Buckhannon 26201				TCH	PBL	12	12	15	24	18	0
002	Garnet Career Ctr Sch of Practical Nsg Mrs Mary Brothers, Coord *Chair's #: (304) 348-6114*	422 Dickinson St Charleston 25301			A	TCH	PBL			Publication withheld			

Explanation of footnotes on page x

School Code	Name of School, Director of Program, and Phone Number	Street Address	City or Town and Zip Code	Footnotes	Type of Program	NLNAC Accreditation as of January 31, 1998	Administrative Control	Financial Support (principal source)	Number of Months in Program	Educational Requirements for Entering Adult Program	Enrollments as of October 15, 1997	Admissions Aug. 1, 1996 - July 31, 1997	Graduations Aug. 1, 1996 - July 31, 1997	Fall Admissions Aug. 1, 1997 - Dec. 31, 1997
010	James Rumsey Tech Inst Mrs Mary Ann Shackelford, Coord *Chair's #: (304) 754-7925 Ext 36*	Rt 6, Box 268	Martinsburg 25401				TCH	PBL	12	12	29	42	27	31
018	Logan-Mingo Sch of PN Mrs Marlene V Newsome, Coord *Chair's #: (304) 752-4687*	Box 1747	Logan 25601				TCH	PBL	12	12	33	34	19	33
019	McDowell Co Voc-Tech Ctr Mrs Francine Kirby, Coord *Chair's #: (304) 436-6180*	Drawer V	Welch 24801				TCH	PVT			Publication withheld			
008	Mercer County Voc-Tech Ctr Ms Sandra Thompson, Coord *Chair's #: (304) 425-7460*	1397 Staffinal Dr	Princeton 24740				TCH	PBL	12	12	26	30	17	30
076	Mineral County Voc Sch of PN Ms Rita Jean Harber, Coord *Chair's #: (304) 788-4240 Ext 17*	600 South Water St	Keyser 26726				TCH	PBL	12	12	18	25	14	0
029	Mingo Co Voc Sch of PN Ms Teresa Anne Carter, Dir *Chair's #: (304) 475-2078*	Rt 2 Box 52-A	Delbarton 25670				TCH	PBL			Publication withheld			
007	Monongalia Co Voc-Tech Ctr Mrs Lynda Overking, Coord *Chair's #: (304) 291-9240 Ext 22*	1000 Mississippi St	Morgantown 26505				TCH	PBL	12	12	28	30	24	30
031	Randoph County Voc Mrs Ruth Caplinger, Coord *Chair's #: (304) 636-9195*	Rt3 Box 246	Elkins 26441				TCH	PBL	12	12	20	25	20	0
023	Region IV Sch of PN Miss Catherine Relihan, Coord *Chair's #: (304) 647-6487*	PO Box 289	Lewisburg 24901				TCH	PBL			Publication withheld			
022	Roane-Jackson Tech Center Ms Donita Gandee, Coord *Chair's #: (304) 372-7335 Ext 39*	4800 Spencer Rd	Leroy 25252				TCH	PBL	12	12	22	28	22	0
020	Summers County Voc Sch Mrs Judith Long, Coord *Chair's #: (304) 466-6040 Ext 128*	116 Main St	Hinton 25951				TCH	PVT	12	12	18	20	16	20
013	United Tech Center Sch of PN Mrs Monica Iaquinta, Facilitator *Chair's #: (304) 624-3284*	Rt 3, Box 43C	Clarksburg 26301				TCH	PBL	12	12	24	27	19	26
003	West Va Northern Comm Coll Dr Regina Jennette, Dir *Chair's #: (304) 233-5900 Ext 4408*	College Sq	Wheeling 26603	7			CC	PBL			Data reported w/AD prog			

School Code	Name of School, Director of Program, and Phone Number	Street Address, City or Town and Zip Code		Footnotes	Type of Program	NLNAC Accreditation as of January 31, 1998	Administrative Control	Financial Support (principal source)	Number of Months in Program	Educational Requirements for Entering Adult Program	Enrollments as of October 15, 1997	Admissions Aug. 1, 1996 - July 31, 1997	Graduations Aug. 1, 1996 - July 31, 1997	Fall Admissions Aug. 1, 1997 - Dec. 31, 1997
	WEST VIRGINIA													
	- Continued													
017	Wood County Vocational School Mrs Carolyn Edwards, Coord *Chair's #: (304) 420-9651 Ext 264*	1515 Blizzard Dr Parkersburg	26101			A	TCH	PBL	12	12	30	28	23	30
024	Wyoming Co Voc Sch Ms Susan Browning, Coord *Chair's #: (304) 732-8050 Ext 105*	HCr 72 Box 200 HCR Pineville	24874				TCH	PBL			Publication withheld			
	WISCONSIN													
	13 Programs in 13 Schools													
017	Blackhawk Tech College Ms Beth Oren, Assoc Dean *Chair's #: (608) 757-7690*	6004 Prairie Rd PO Box 5009 Janesville	53547	2			TCH	PBL			Publication withheld			
013	Chippewa Valley Tech College Ms M Dickens-Grosskopf , Dir *Chair's #: (715) 833-6419*	620 W Clairemont Ave Eau Claire	54701				TCH	PBL	9	12	9	19	5	9
003	Fox Valley Tech College Mrs Ardythe Korpela, Dept Chair *Chair's #: (920) 735-5664*	1825 N Bluemound Dr Appleton	54913				TCH	PBL	12	10	34	78	37	30
015	Gateway Tech Coll Mrs Kathleen Russ, Dean *Chair's #: (414) 656-6934*	3520 30th Ave Kenosha	53144				TCH	PBL	9	12	50	40	39	20
012	Lakeshore Tech College Ms Nancy Kaprelian, Dean *Chair's #: (920) 458-4183 Ext 0180*	1290 North Ave Cleveland	53015	7			TCH	PBL			Data reported w/AD prog			
004	Madison Area Tech College Ms Alda Preston, Assoc Dean *Chair's #: (608) 246-6014*	3550 Anderson St Madison	53704			A	TCH	PBL	11	12	58	65	49	44
002	Milwaukee Area Tech College PN Progr Dr Mary E Eiche, Assoc Dean *Chair's #: (414) 297-6241*	700 W State St Milwaukee	53233			A	TCH	PBL			Publication withheld			
007	Moraine Park Tech College Mrs Wendy McCulloch, Dir *Chair's #: (414) 335-5720*	700 Gould St Beaver Dam	53916			A	CC	PBL	9	12	36	40	30	19
008	NE Wisconsin Tech College Dr Judith Mix, Assoc Dean *Chair's #: (920) 498-5482*	2740 W Mason St Box 19042 Green Bay	54307				TCH	PBL	11	12	24	23	20	24
014	SW Wisconsin Tech College Ms Sharon Selleck-Lehman, Dean *Chair's #: (608) 822-3262 Ext 2151*	1800 Bronson Blvd Fennimore	53809			A	TCH	PBL	10	12	20	23	16	20

Explanation of footnotes on page x

School Code	Name of School, Director of Program, and Phone Number	Street Address City or Town and Zip Code		Footnotes	Type of Program	NLNAC Accreditation as of January 31, 1998	Administrative Control	Financial Support (principal source)	Number of Months in Program	Educational Requirements for Entering Adult Program	Enrollments as of October 15, 1997	Admissions Aug. 1, 1996 - July 31, 1997	Graduations Aug. 1, 1996 - July 31, 1997	Fall Admissions Aug. 1, 1997 - Dec. 31, 1997
	WISCONSIN													
	- Continued													
011	Waukesha County Tech College Dr Kitty Gotham, Assoc Dean Chair's #: (414) 691-5368	800 Main St Pewaukee	53072	6			TCH	PBL			Publication withheld			
016	Western Wisconsin Tech Coll Ms Donna Haggard, Chair Chair's #: (608) 785-9186	304 N 6th St La Crosse	54602	6			TCH	PBL			Publication withheld			
	WYOMING													
	5 Programs in 5 Schools													
001	Casper College Mrs Judith Turner, Chair Chair's #: (307) 268-2233	125 College Dr Casper	82601				CC	PBL			Publication withheld			
003	Laramie County Comm College Ms Jan Freudenthal, Coord Chair's #: (307) 778-1133	1400 E College Dr Cheyenne	82007	7		A	CC	PBL			Data reported w\AD prog			
007	Northern Wyoming Comm College PN P Mrs Nancy Larmer, Director Chair's #: (307) 686-1358 Ext 227	750 W 8th Suite 1 Gillette	82716				CC	PBL	9	12	0	0	13	0
005	Northwest College Mr William Clinton, Dir Chair's #: (307) 754-6479	231 W 6th Powell	82435	7		A	CC	PBL			Data reported w/ AD prog			
004	Sheridan College Dr Michael Enos, Dir Chair's #: (307) 674-6446 Ext 6153	Sheridan	82801	7		A	CC	PBL			Data reported w/AD prog			

SUMMARY TABLES

NEW SCHOOLS*
(Between October 16, 1996 and October 15, 1997)

STATE	SCHOOL OF NURSING -L.P.N./L.V.N.	CITY or TOWN	TYPE OF PROGRAM
AK	University of Alaska -Nursing Department	Fairbanks	Adult
CA	Marian College	Los Angeles	Adult
FL	Academy for Practical Nursing	West Palm Beach	Adult
	Gadsden Tech. Institute	Quincy	Adult
MI	Bay Mills Community College	Brinley	Adult
	Grand Rapids Educational Centers	Grand Rapids	Adult
MO	Moberly Area Community College	Mexico	Adult
PR	Atenas College	Manati	Adult
	Metro College	Caguas	Adult
	Medical Tech. College	Yauco	Adult
	John Dewey College	Carolina	Adult
	Universidad Interamericana	Arecibo	Adult
	Ponce Paramedical College	Ponce	Adult
TN	Baptist Memorial College of Health Sciences	Memphis	Adult
TX	Austin Community College	Fredericksburg	Adult
WA	Grays Harbor College	Aberdeen	Adult
VA	Dabney S. Lancaster Community College	Clifton Forge	Adult
	Virginia Western Community College	Roanoke	Adult
WI	Blackhawk Tech. College	Janesville	Adult
MA	Montachussett RVTS	Fitchburg	Adult

*Complete information about each new school can be located in the body of this report under each new school.

CLOSED SCHOOLS
(Between October 16, 1996 and October 15, 1997)

STATE	SCHOOL OF NURSING -L.P.N./L.V.N.	CITY or TOWN	TYPE OF PROGRAM	NLN ACCREDITATION STATUS	ADMINISTRATIVE CONTROL	FINANCIAL SUPPORT	GRADUATIONS: Aug.1, 1996 – July 31, 1997
CO	Pikes Peak Community College	Colorado Springs	Adult	-	CC	PBL	-
FL	Orange Tech Ed. Center	Winter Garden	Adult	-	TCH	PBL	-
GA	Kinderlin Tech. Institute	Gordon	Adult	-	TCH	PVT	-
MD	Johnston School of PN — Union Memorial Hospital	Baltimore	Adult	A	HSP	PVT	-
MA	Tewksbury Hospital	Tewksbury	Adult	A	HSP	PBL	-
MO	Applied Technology Services/N. County	Florissant	Adult	-	TCH	PBL	-
	Mexico Public School	Mexico	Adult	-	TCH	PBL	-
NC	Rowan Cabarrus Community College	Salisbury	Adult	-	CC	PBL	-
PA	School District of Philadelphia/James Martin	Philadelphia	Adult	A	TCH	PBL	-
PR	Instituto de Educacion Universal	Sabana Seca	Adult	-	TCH	PVT	-
	Instituto de Educacion Universal	Carolina	Adult	-	SEC	PBL	-
	Instituto de Educacion	Hato Rey	Adult	-	SEC	PBL	-
TN	Reginal Medical Center	Memphis	Adult	-	HSP	PBL	-
	Science Hill Tech. Center	Johnson City	Adult	-	SEC	PVT	-
TX	Howard College	Fredericksburg	Adult	-	CC	PBL	-
VA	Triplett Business and Tech. Institute	Mount Jackson	Adult	-	TCH	PBL	-
VI	Raphael O. Wheatley Skills Center	St. Thomas	Adult	-	GOV	PBL	-

DIRECTORY OF
BOARDS OF NURSING

DIRECTORY OF
BOARDS OF NURSING

Judi Crume, Exec. Off.
AL Board of Nursing
P.O. Box 303900
Montgomery, Alabama 36130-3900
Tel (334) 242-4060

Dorothy Fulton, Exec. Admin.
Alaska Board of Nursing
3601 "C" St., Suite 722
Anchorage, Alaska 99503
Tel (907) 269-8161

Etenauga Lam Yuen Lutu, Exec. Dir.
Health Services Regulatory Bd.
LBJ Tropical Med. Ctr.
Pago Pago, American Samoa 96799
Tel (684) 633-5995

Joey Ridenour, Exec. Dir.
Arizona State Board of Nursing
1651 E. Morton, Suite 150
Phoenix, Arizona 85020
Tel (602) 331-8111

Faith Fields, Exec. Dir.
Arkansas State Board of Nursing
1123 South Univ., Suite 800
Little Rock, Arkansas 72204
Tel (501) 686-2700

Teresa Bello Jones, Exec. Off.
Bd. of VN & Psych. Tech. Examiners
2535 Capitol Oaks Dr., Suite 205
Sacramento, California 95833-2919
Tel (916) 263-7840

Karen Brumley, Admin.
Colorado State Board of Nursing
1560 Broadway, Suite 670
Denver, Colorado 80202-2410
Tel (303) 894-2819

Wendy Furmisa, Supr.
Department of Public Health
Board of Examiners for Nsg.
410 Capitol Ave.
P.O. Box 340308
Hartford, Connecticut 06134-0308
Tel (860) 509-7400

Iva J. Boardman, Exec. Dir.
Delaware Board of Nursing
Cannon Bldg., P.O. Box 1401
Dover, Delaware 19901
Tel (302) 739-4522, Ext. 217

Barbara W. Hagans, Contact Rep.
District of Columbia Board of Nursing
614 H St., N.W.
Washington, D.C. 20013
Tel (202) 727-7856

Marilyn A. Bloss, Exec. Dir.
Florida State Board of Nursing
4080 Woodcock Dr., Suite 202
Jacksonville, Florida 32207
Tel (904) 858-6940

Janet M. Starr, Nsg. Educ. Consultant
Georgia Board of Examiners of
Lic. Practical Nurse
166 Pryor St., N.W., Suite 300
Atlanta, Georgia 30303
Tel (404) 656-3921

Teo-Fila Cruz, Exec. Dir.
Guam Board of Nurse Examiners
P.O. Box 2816
Agana, Guam 96910
Tel (671) 734-7295

Kathleen Yokouchi, Exec. Off.
Hawaii Board of Nursing
Box 3469
Honolulu, Hawaii 99503
Tel (808) 586-2695

Sandra Evans, Asst. Exec. Dir.
Idaho State Board of Nursing
P.O. Box 83720
Boise, Idaho 83720-0061
Tel (208) 334-3110

Elizabeth Cleinmark, Acting Coord.
Department of Professional Regulation
320 W. Washington St.
Springfield, Illinois 62786
Tel (217) 785-9465

Gina Voorhies, Dir.
Indiana State Board of Nursing
402 W. Washington St.
Indianapolis, Indiana 46204
Tel (317) 233-4405

Lorinda Inman, Exec. Dir.
Iowa Board of Nursing
1223 E. Court Ave.
Des Moines, Iowa 50319
Tel (515) 281-4828

Pat Johnson, Exec. Admin.
Kansas State Board of Nursing
900 SW Jackson St., Suite 551S
Topeka, Kansas 66612-1256
Tel (785) 296-3782

Sharon M. Weisenbeck, Exec. Dir.
Kentucky Board of Nursing
312 Whittington Pky., Suite 300
Louisville, Kentucky 40222-5172
Tel (502) 329-7000, ext. 235

Terry L. Demarcay, Exec. Dir.
Louisiana State Bd. of PN Examiners
3421 N Causeway Blvd., Suite 203
Metairie, Louisiana 70002-5791
Tel (504) 838-5791

Jean C. Caron, Exec. Dir.
Maine State Board of Nursing
35 Anthony Ave. St. House Sta. 158
Augusta, Maine 04333-0158
Tel (207) 287-1133

Donna Dorsey, Exec. Dir.
Maryland Board of Nursing
4140 Patterson Ave.
Baltimore, Maryland 21215-2254
Tel (410) 764-5124

Theresa M. Bonanno, Exec. Dir.
Board of Registration in Nursing
100 Cambridge St., Room 150
Boston, Massachusetts 02202
Tel (617) 727-3060

Mary A. Vanden Bosch, Nurse Consultant
Michigan Board of Nursing
P.O. Box 30018, 611 West Ottawa
Lansing, Michigan 48909
Tel (517) 373-4674

Joyce M. Schowalter, Exec. Dir.
Minnesota Board of Nursing
2829 University Ave., SE #500
Minneapolis, Minnesota 55114-3253
Tel (612) 617-2294

Gail Caraway, Supv.
Health Occupations Ed.,
Div. of Vocational Ed.
Dept. of Education, P.O. Box 771
Jackson, Mississippi 39205
Tel (601) 359-3461

Florence Stillman, Exec. Dir.
Missouri State Board of Nursing
3605 Missouri Blvd., Box 656
Jefferson City, Missouri 65102-0656
Tel (573) 751-0080

Dianne Wickham, Exec. Dir.
Montana State Board of Nursing
111 Jackson, Arcade Bldg.
Helena, Montana 59620-0513
Tel (406) 444-2071

Charlene Kelley, Assoc. Dir.
Bureau of Examining Board
P.O. Box 95007
Lincoln, Nebraska 68509
Tel (402) 471-4917

Kathy Apple, Exec. Dir.
Nevada State Board of Nursing
4335 S. Industrial Rd. #420
Las Vegas, Nevada 89103
Tel (702) 739-1575

Doris G. Nuttelman, Exec. Dir.
State Board of Nursing
Div. of Public Hlth, 6 Hazen Dr.
Concord, New Hampshire 03301
Tel (603) 271-2323

Harriet Johnson, Asst. Exec. Dir.
New Jersey Board of Nursing
P.O. Box 45010
Newark, New Jersey 07101
Tel (973) 504-6430

Nancy L. Twigg, Exec. Dir.
New Mexico Board of Nursing
4206 Louisiana NE, Suite A
Albuquerque, New Mexico 87109
Tel (505) 841-8340

Milene A. Sower, Exec. Sec.
New York State Board for Nursing
The Cultural Center, Room 3023
Albany, New York 12230
Tel (518) 486-2967

Carol A. Osman, Exec. Dir.
NC Board of Nursing
P.O. Box 2129
Raleigh, North Carolina 27602
Tel (919) 782-3211

Ida H. Rigley, Exec. Dir.
North Dakota Board of Nursing
919 S. 7th St., Suite 504
Bismarck, North Dakota 58504-5881
Tel (701) 328-9777

Dorothy Fiorino, Exec. Dir.
Ohio Board of Nursing
77 S. High St., 17th Floor
Columbus, Ohio 43266-0316
Tel (614) 466-9800

Sulinda Moffett, Exec. Dir.
Oklahoma Board of Nursing
2915 N. Classen Blvd., Suite 524
Oklahoma City, Oklahoma 73106
Tel (405) 525-2076

Joan Bouchard, Exec. Dir.
Oregon State Board of Nursing
800 N.E. Oregon St., #25
Portland, Oregon 97232
Tel (503) 731-4745

Miriam H. Limo, Exec. Sec.
Pennsylvania State Board of Nurses
P.O. Box 2649
Harrisburg, Pennsylvania 17105
Tel (717) 772-8547

Osvaldo Feliú Miranda, Dir.
General Council on Education
P.O. Box 195429
San Juan, Puerto Rico 00919-5429
Tel (787) 764-0101

Patricia Molloy, Dir.
Board of Nsg. Educ. & Nurse Registration
3 Capitol Hill
Providence, Rhode Island 02908-5097
Tel (401) 277-2827

Patricia Durgin, Admin.
State Board of Nursing for South Carolina
220 Executive Center Dr., Suite 220
Columbia, South Carolina 29210
Tel (803) 896-4529

Gloria Damgaard, Educ. Specialist
South Dakota Board of Nursing
3307 South Lincoln
Sioux Falls, South Dakota 57105
Tel (605) 367-5940

Elizabeth J. Lund, Exec. Dir.
TN Board of Nursing
425 Fifth Ave. N.
Nashville, Tennessee 37247-1010
Tel (615) 532-5166

Marjorie A. Bronk, Exec. Dir.
Board of Vocational Nurse Examiners
333 Guadalupe St., Suite 3-100
Austin, Texas 78701
Tel (512) 305-8100, Ext. 215

Laura Poe, Exec. Admin.
Utah State Board of Nursing
160 E. 300 South, Box 45805
Salt Lake City, Utah 84145
Tel (801) 530-6789

Anita Ristau, Exec. Dir.
Vermont Board of Nursing
Licensing and Registration Div.
109 State St.
Montpelier, Vermont 05602
Tel (802) 828-2396

Winifred Garfield, Exec. Dir.
Virgin Islands Board of Nurse Licensure
P.O. Box 4247
Charolotte Amalie, Virgin Islands 00803
Tel (809) 776-7397

Nancy K. Durrett, Exec. Dir.
Virginia Board of Nursing
6606 W. Broad St., 4th Floor
Richmond, Virginia 23230-1717
Tel (804) 662-9951

Patty Hayes, Exec. Dir.
WA St. Nsg. Care Quality Assur. Commission
1300 Quince, P.O. Box 47864
Olympia, Washington 98504-7864
Tel (360) 664-4208

Nancy R. Wilson, Exec. Sec.
WV State Board of Examiners for Licensed PN
101 Dee Dr.
Charleston, West Virginia 25311-1688
Tel (304) 348-3572

Thomas A. Neumann, Admin. Off.
Wisconsin Dept. of Regulation & Licensing
P.O. Box 8935
Madison, Wisconsin 53708-8935
Tel (608) 267-2357

Mary Shaper, Interim Exec. Dir.
State of Wyoming Board of Nursing
2301 Central Ave., Barrett Bldg.
Cheyenne, Wyoming 82002
Tel (307) 777-6127